MRCP 1
Best of Five
Multiple Choice Revision Book

Second Edition

Khalid Binymin
MBChB MSc FRCP
Consultant Physician and Rheumatologist
Honorary Lecturer at Liverpool University

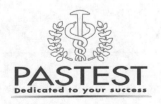

PASTEST
Dedicated to your success

© 2005 PASTEST LTD
Egerton Court
Parkgate Estate
Knutsford
Cheshire
WA16 8DX

Telephone: 01565 752000

First Edition 2002
Second Edition 2005

ISBN: 190462748X

A catalogue record for this book is available from the British Library.

The information contained within this book was obtained by the author from reliable sources. However, while every effort has been make to ensure its accuracy, no responsibility for loss, damage or injury occasioned to any person acting or refraining from action as a result of information contained herein can be accepted by the publishers or author.

PasTest Revision Books and Intensive Courses

PasTest has been established in the field of postgraduate medical education since 1972, providing revision books and intensive study courses for doctors preparing for their professional examinations.

Books and courses are available for the following specialties:

MRCGP, MRCP Parts 1 and 2, MRCPCH Parts 1 and 2, MRCPsych, MRCS, MRCOG Parts 1 and 2, DRCOG, DCH, FRCA, PLAB Parts 1 and 2.

For further details contact:

PasTest, Freepost, Knutsford, Cheshire WA16 7BR
Tel: 01565 752000   Fax: 01565 650264
www.pastest.co.uk   enquires@pastest.co.uk

Text prepared by Vision Typesetting Ltd, Manchester
Printed and bound in the UK by MPG Books, Cornwall

CONTENTS

iii

ACKNOWLEDGEMENTS

S Almond
Consultant, Acute Medical Unit, Royal Liverpool Hospital, Liverpool.

N Kennedy
Consultant Physician in Infectious Diseases, Monklands Hospital, Airdrie.

B Maher
Senior Registrar in Medicine, Royal Liverpool Hospital, Liverpool.

P Murray
Specialist Registrar in Respiratory Medicine, North East Thames
(Rotation), London.

H Paynter
Formerly Specialist Registrar in Renal Medicine, Gloucestershire Royal
Hospital, Gloucester.

K Smyth
Consultant Ophthalmologist, Royal Bolton Hospital, Bolton.

A Wade
Senior Lecturer in Medical Statistics, Department of Epidemiology and
Public Health, Institute of Child Health, London.

PREFACE

Following the success of the revision book – *MRCP 1 Best of Five Multiple Choice Revision Book* – I was given the opportunity to write the second edition of this best-seller to capture the new advances in medicine and to incorporate the actual examination format. In this new improved edition, clinical scenarios are added to all questions where possible and new questions are added to cover many recurring themes in the MRCP examinations. Answers include full detailed explanations enabling the reader to develop their understanding of each condition or topic.

The second edition aims to test the widest breadth of the candidate's knowledge. More than 300 questions offer effective exam practice and guide candidates through their revision and exam technique. The book consists of 16 chapters that comply with and satisfy the Royal College of Physicians' curriculum for the MRCP Part 1 examination. The questions are stimulating and challenging. This title promotes the building of a good level of knowledge and confidence essential for all candidates taking the examination.

I hope you have as much pleasure in reading it as I did in preparing it.

Dr Khalid Binymin
MBChB MSc FRCP
Honorary lecturer at Liverpool University

NORMAL VALUES

Blood, serum and plasma

Haematology

Haemoglobin	12.5–14.5 g/dl
Mean corpuscular volume (MCV)	80–96 fl
Mean corpuscular haemoglobin (MCH)	28–32 pg
Mean corpuscular haemoglobin concentration (MCHC)	32–35 g/dl
White cell count (WCC)	$4–11 \times 10^9/l$
Differential WCC: neutrophils	$1.5–7 \times 10^9/l$
lymphocytes	$1.5–4 \times 10^9/l$
eosinophils	$0.04–0.4 \times 10^9/l$
Platelet count	$150–400 \times 10^9/l$
Reticulocyte count	$50–100 \times 10^9/l$
Prothrombin time (PT)	12–17 s
Activated partial thromboplastin time (APTT)	30–40 s
Thrombin time (TT)	14–22 s
Fibrinogen	2–5 g/l
Fibrinogen degradation products (FDP)	<10 µg/ml
International normalised ratio (INR)	<1.4
Iron (Fe^{2+})	14–29 µmol/l
Total iron-binding capacity (TIBC)	45–72 µmol/l
Ferritin	15–300 µg/l
Vitamin B_{12}	120–700 pmol/l
Folate (serum)	2.0–11.0 µg/l

Red cell folate	160–640 µg/l
Erythrocyte sedimentation rate (ESR)	<12 mm/(1st) hour
Plasma viscosity	1.5–1.72 cP

Immunology/Rheumatology

C-reactive protein (CRP)	<5mg/l
IgG	6.0–13.0 g/l
IgM	0.4–2.5 g/l
IgA	0.8–3.0 g/l
β_2-Microglobulin	<3 mg/l

Endocrinology

Fasting glucose	3.0–6.0 mmol/l
Hb A_{1c}	3.8–6.4%
Thyroid stimulating hormone (TSH)	0.3–4.0 mU/l
Thyroxine (T4)	58–174 nmol/l
Free T4 (FT4)	10–24 pmol/l
Parathyroid hormone (PTH)	0.9–5.4 pmol/l
Prolactin	<360 mU/l

Biochemistry

Sodium (Na^+)	137–144 mmol/l
Potassium (K^+)	3.5–4.9 mmol/l
Chloride	95–107 mmol/l
Anion gap	12–16 mmol/l
Urea	2.5–7.5 mmol/l
Creatinine	60–110 µmol/l
Calcium (Ca^{2+}), corrected	2.25–2.70 mmol/l
Phosphate	0.8–1.4 mmol/l
Creatine kinase (CK)	<120 U/l
Uric acid	0–0.43 mmol/l
Copper	12–26 µmol/l
Magnesium	0.75–1.05 mmol/l
Lactate	0.6–1.8 mmol/l
Caeruloplasmin	200–350 mg/l
Amylase	60–180 U/l
Plasma osmolality	278–305 mosmol/kg

Alanine aminotransferase (ALT)	5–35 U/l
Aspartate aminotransferase (AST)	1–31 U/l
Alkaline phosphatase (ALP)	45–105 U/l
Lactate dehydrogenase (LDH)	10–250 U/l
γ-Glutamyl transferase (GGT)	4–35 U/l
	(<50 U/l in men)
Bilirubin (total)	1–22 μmol/l
Bilirubin (direct, or conjugated)	0–3.4 μmol/l
Total protein	61–76 g/l
Albumin	37–49 g/l
α-Fetoprotein (AFP)	<10–20 μg/l (kU/l)
Cholesterol	<5.2 mmol/l
Triglyceride (fasting)	0.45–1.69 mmol/l

Blood gases

pH	7.36–7.44
PaO_2	11.3–12.6 kPa
$PaCO_2$	4.7–6.0 kPa
Bicarbonate	20–28 mmol/l
Base excess	±2 mmol/l

Therapeutic drug levels

Digoxin (≥6 h post-dose)	1–2 μg/l
Gentamicin	5–7 μg/ml
Lithium	0.4–1.0 mol/l

Urine

Albumin	<30 mg/24 h
Albumin/creatinine ratio (random sample)	< 2.5 mg/mmol
Total protein	< 0.2 g/24 h
Glomerular filtration rate (GFR)	70–140 ml/min
Osmolality	350–1000 mosmol/kg

Cerebrospinal fluid (CSF)

Opening pressure	5–18 cmH$_2$O

Total protein		0.15–0.45 g/l
Glucose		3.3–4.4 mmol/l
Cell count		<5 cells/mm^3
Differential cell count:	lymphocytes	60–70%
	monocytes	30–50%
	neutrophils	none

The Questions

Chapter 1
BASIC SCIENCES
Questions

1.1 **Which one of the following is the main function of the Golgi apparatus?**

☐ A   It packages molecules into vesicles that can be transported out of a cell
☐ B   It produces most of the cell's energy requirements
☐ C   It is responsible for bacterial phagocytosis
☐ D   It regulates cell reproduction
☐ E   Protein synthesis

1.2 **Which one of the following is the definition of 'apoptosis'?**

☐ A   Programmed cell death
☐ B   Phagocytosis of nuclear material
☐ C   Forward movement of the eyeball
☐ D   Inflammation of the tendon sheath
☐ E   Cell necrosis

1.3 **Which one of the following is true with regard to cytokines?**

☐ A   Cytokines are produced exclusively by cells of the immune system
☐ B   Interleukin 6 (IL-6) enhances albumin synthesis by the liver
☐ C   Interleukin 2 (IL-2) is derived from wandering macrophages
☐ D T_H1 cells regulate allergic reactions and antibody production
☐ E   Transforming growth factor β (TGF-β) inhibits the production of other cytokines

Answers on pages 135–136   3

1.4   Which one of the following statements about seminal fluid is true?

☐   A   Semen is produced in the seminal vesicles and stored in the testes

☐   B   In a human, complete maturation of spermatozoa takes approximately 3 hours

☐   C   Up to 70% of the spermatozoa in an ejaculate are abnormal

☐   D   The spermatozoon concentration may be temporarily suppressed by fever

☐   E   Sildenafil (Viagra®) doubles the sperm count 3 months after the initiation of treatment

1.5   Which one of the following factors inhibits the release of renin?

☐   A   Assumption of the erect posture

☐   B   Overactive sympathetic adrenergic neurones

☐   C   Salt depletion

☐   D   Prostaglandins

☐   E   Angiotensin II

1.6   Which one of the following muscles in the hand is supplied by the median nerve?

☐   A   Lateral two interossei

☐   B   Abductor pollicis brevis

☐   C   Medial two lumbricals

☐   D   Flexor pollicis longus

☐   E   Extensor pollicis

1.7   Which one of the following statements is true regarding vasopressin?

☐   A   It is synthesised in the posterior pituitary

☐   B   It makes the proximal convoluted tubules more permeable to hypotonic fluid

☐   C   It increases the concentrations of circulating factor VIII and von Willebrand factor

☐   D   It inhibits the release of adrenocorticotrophic hormone (ACTH) from the pituitary

☐   E   It induces vasodilatation in splanchnic vessels

1.8 Osteopetrosis (marble bone disease) is characterised by sclerosis and obliteration of the bone marrow due to abnormal function of which one of the following cell types?

☐ A Osteoblasts
☐ B Osteoclasts
☐ C Chondrocytes
☐ D Synoviocytes
☐ E Macrophages

1.9 Which one of the following statements about physiological acclimatisation to high altitude is true?

☐ A It starts at an altitude of 1000 feet
☐ B The plasma volume increases
☐ C The haematocrit is reduced
☐ D There is increased renal excretion of bicarbonate
☐ E There is pulmonary hypoventilation

1.10 A 50-year-old woman is referred with general lethargy and excessive fatigue. The serum sodium is 117 mmol/l. You suspect that she has syndrome of inappropriate antidiuretic hormone secretion (SIADH). Which one of the following findings would be most typical of this syndrome?

☐ A Urinary sodium excretion of 10 mmol/l
☐ B Urine osmolality of 120 mosmol/kg
☐ C Plasma osmolality of 300 mosmol/kg
☐ D Serum potassium concentration of 3 mmol/l
☐ E Urine output of 2 litres/24 hours

1.11 Which one of the following is most likely to increase during exercise?

☐ A Peripheral vascular resistance
☐ B Pulmonary vascular resistance
☐ C Stroke volume
☐ D Diastolic pressure
☐ E Venous compliance

1.12   Which one of the following statements about hyponatraemia is accurate?

☐   A   In heart failure it is associated with a poor prognosis
☐   B   In liver cirrhosis it is often due to increased renal loss of sodium
☐   C   When associated with hypo-osmolarity, paraproteinaemia should be considered
☐   D   In the presence of low urea and low serum potassium levels, it is suggestive of Addison's disease
☐   E   Confusion and coma often ensue when serum sodium approaches 125 mmol/l

1.13   Which one of the following is higher at the apex of the lung than at the base of the lung when a person is standing?

☐   A $\dot{V}/\dot{Q}$ ratio
☐   B   Ventilation
☐   C Pa_{CO_2}
☐   D   Compliance
☐   E   Blood flow

1.14   The primary neurochemical disturbance in idiopathic Parkinson's disease involves which one of the following?

☐   A   Noradrenaline (norepinephrine)
☐   B   Dopamine
☐   C   γ-Aminobutyric acid (GABA)
☐   D   Substance P
☐   E   Adrenaline (epinephrine)

1.15   Which one of the following pathological features is pathognomonic of the disease it is listed with?

☐   A   Reed–Sternberg cells in Hodgkin's disease
☐   B   Aschoff nodules in rheumatic fever
☐   C   Charcot–Leyden crystals in sputum from a patient with asthma
☐   D   Alcoholic hyaline (Mallory body) from a liver biopsy specimen in alcoholic liver disease
☐   E   Non-caseating granuloma in sarcoidosis

1.16   The secretion of growth hormone is increased by which one of the following?

☐   A   Hyperglycaemia
☐   B   Exercise
☐   C   Somatostatin
☐   D   Growth hormone
☐   E   Free fatty acids

1.17   As a hormone, steroid produces its catabolic effect on human body cells via which one of the following?

☐   A   Cell membrane receptors
☐   B   Increased synthesis of cholesterol
☐   C   Cyclic AMP
☐   D   Intracellular protein kinase
☐   E   The nucleus

1.18   Which one of the following statements regarding cerebrospinal fluid (CSF) is true?

☐   A   It is absorbed by the choroid plexus
☐   B   It circulates in the epidural space
☐   C   It has a lower glucose concentration than plasma
☐   D   It has a higher protein concentration than plasma
☐   E   It diffuses along the nerves back into the blood circulation

1.19   Which one of the following inhibits aldosterone secretion?

☐   A   Angiotensin II
☐   B   ACTH
☐   C   Hyponatraemia
☐   D   Hyperkalaemia
☐   E   Renin

Answers on pages 139–141

1.20   Which one of the following statements about tumour necrosis factor (TNF) is true?

☐   A   It inhibits angiogenesis (hence its prominent anti-tumour activity)
☐   B   It promotes inflammation
☐   C   It neutralises adhesion molecules
☐   D   It is produced primarily by activated B lymphocytes
☐   E   Anti-TNF-α therapies have been withdrawn as they doubled the risk of solid tumours

1.21   Vasoconstriction in response to hypoxia occurs in which one of the following vascular beds?

☐   A   Hepatic
☐   B   Cerebral
☐   C   Cutaneous
☐   D   Renal
☐   E   Coronary

1.22   Which one of the following statements about the diaphragm is true?

☐   A   It is composed of smooth involuntary muscle and a central tendon
☐   B   It is innervated by the long thoracic nerve
☐   C   The left hemidiaphragm is normally higher than the right one
☐   D   When paralysed it becomes flattened
☐   E   Hiccup is caused by spasmodic contraction of the diaphragm

1.23   A 69-year-old man presents with acute confusion. He has lost 8 kg in weight in the last 2 months. Blood tests reveal a serum calcium concentration of 3 mmol/l and a significantly elevated parathyroid hormone-related peptide (PTHrP) level. Which one of the following tumour cell types is most probably responsible for this disorder?

☐   A   Neuroendocrine
☐   B   Squamous
☐   C   Large cell
☐   D   Mesenchymal
☐   E   Columnar

1.24 **Which one of the following statements about the complement system is true?**

☐ A IgA activates the classical complement pathway

☐ B Hereditary angio-oedema is associated with C1 complement deficiency

☐ C Hypocomplementaemia is often an early feature of renal disease in scleroderma

☐ D Homozygous C2 deficiency is associated with systemic lupus erythematosus

☐ E Homozygous C7 deficiency is associated with increased susceptibility to HIV infections

1.25 **Leptin is a hormone responsible for regulating fat mass in the body. Which one of the following statements about this hormone is true?**

☐ A It is secreted by the pancreas

☐ B It acts directly on adipocytes in the subcutaneous tissue and causes proliferation of fat cells

☐ C The vast majority of obese individuals have markedly elevated plasma leptin concentrations

☐ D It enhances appetite

☐ E It suppresses energy expenditure

1.26 **Which one of the following statements is true with regard to a high potassium intake?**

☐ A It raises the systolic blood pressure by 5–10 mmHg

☐ B It increases the risk of stroke

☐ C It reduces urinary calcium excretion, which reduces the risk of kidney stones

☐ D It promotes bone demineralisation

☐ E It lowers a high blood cholesterol

1.27 **Which one of the following represents the recommended daily dietary intake of calcium and vitamin D in the treatment of established osteoporosis?**

☐ A 800 mg/day of calcium, 100 units/day of vitamin D
☐ B 1500 mg/day of calcium, 400–800 units/day of vitamin D
☐ C 1200 mg/day of calcium, 200–400 units/day of vitamin D
☐ D 900 mg/day of calcium, 200 units/day of vitamin D
☐ E 1800 mg/day of calcium, 800–1000 units/day of vitamin D

1.28 **Which one of the following statements about immunoglobulins is true?**

☐ A IgA immunoglobulins cross the placenta
☐ B IgG has the highest molecular weight
☐ C IgM has the highest concentration in plasma
☐ D All immunoglobulins except for IgG are synthesised in the liver
☐ E Levels are typically normal in DiGeorge syndrome

1.29 **Which one of the following effects of selective inhibition of cyclooxygenase-2 (COX-2) enzyme is not as prominent as it is in selective inhibition of cyclooxygenase-1 (COX-1)?**

☐ A Anti-inflammatory
☐ B Antiplatelet
☐ C Analgesic
☐ D Sodium retention
☐ E Bronchospasm

1.30 A 70-year-old diabetic woman presents with a gradual decline in her general health and increasing drowsiness. She is recovering from a recent chest infection. The blood tests show: glucose 33 mmol/l, urea 12 mmol/l, sodium 150 mmol/l, potassium 4.5 mmol/l, haemoglobin 11 g/dl. You suspect hyperosmolar non-ketotic diabetic coma. Which one of the following is the measured plasma osmolality?

☐ A 345 mosmol/kg
☐ B 325 mosmol/kg
☐ C 195 mosmol/kg
☐ D 185 mosmol/kg
☐ E 183 mosmol/kg

Chapter 2

CARDIOLOGY

Questions

2.1 A 55-year-old man is admitted to the Coronary Care Unit with severe central chest pain. The troponin I was significantly raised. The 12-lead ECG shows a Q wave and ST elevation in leads II, III and aVF. Occlusion of which one of the following coronary arteries is responsible for this patient's presentation?

☐ A Right
☐ B Left anterior descending
☐ C Circumflex
☐ D Main stem
☐ E Diagonal

2.2 A 30-year-old woman is having a pre-employment assessment when wide splitting of the second heart sound is noted. Which one of the following disorders is associated with this physical sign?

☐ A Atrial septal defect (ASD)
☐ B Aortic stenosis
☐ C Left bundle branch block (LBBB)
☐ D Type B Wolff–Parkinson–White (WPW) syndrome
☐ E Patent ductus arteriosus (PDA)

Answers on page 147

2.3   A 20-year-old man presents with reduced exercise tolerance and easy fatiguability. His upper arm blood pressure is higher than that in the lower limb. Rib notching and a 'figure 3' sign are identified on a plain chest X-ray. Which one of the following statements is most accurate regarding coarctation of the aorta?

☐   A   The coarctation is proximal to the origin of the left subclavian artery if the right arm blood pressure is significantly higher than that in the left arm

☐   B   A continuous murmur over the thoracic spine usually originates from extensive collaterals

☐   C   Rib notching on plain chest X-ray can be identified as early as 3 months after birth

☐   D   Atrial septal defect (ASD) is the commonest associated congenital abnormality

☐   E   The risk of subacute bacterial endocarditis is low and antibiotic prophylaxis is seldom required

2.4   Which one of the following is characteristic of atrial myxoma?

☐   A   It usually originates in the right atrium
☐   B   Fragments of tumour break off easily and grow in peripheral sites
☐   C   Echocardiogram is diagnostic in most cases
☐   D   The clinical signs can mimic severe mitral regurgitation
☐   E   Recurrence is frequent, even after successful surgical removal of the tumour

2.5 A 60-year-old woman is referred for urgent investigation of a rapid decline in general health, low-grade fever and weight loss. She is known to have developed a murmur following acute rheumatic fever as a teenager. Blood culture is positive for *Streptococcus viridans*. Which one of the following statements regarding this disorder is true?

- [ ] A The risk of infection is higher for mitral valve lesions than it is for aortic valve lesions
- [ ] B Q fever is the most common cause of culture-negative endocarditis
- [ ] C If *Streptococcus bovis* endocarditis is diagnosed, a thorough investigation of the colon is indicated
- [ ] D *Staphylococcus aureus* is frequently isolated in early prosthetic valve endocarditis
- [ ] E Prophylaxis for endocarditis is probably not required to cover cystoscopy

2.6 A 68-year-old man is referred because of increasing shortness of breath. The 12-lead ECG shows a short QT interval. This abnormality is a complication of which one of the following?

- [ ] A Quinidine therapy
- [ ] B Hypokalaemia
- [ ] C Tricyclic antidepressant therapy
- [ ] D Amiodarone therapy
- [ ] E Digoxin therapy

2.7 A 20-year-old drug addict is admitted to the Intensive Care Unit with fever, clouding of consciousness and increasing shortness of breath. The echocardiogram shows vegetations and the blood culture is positive from two bottles. Which one of the following is true of this type of bacterial endocarditis?

- [ ] A *Staphylococcus aureus* is the most frequent causative agent
- [ ] B The echocardiogram is often normal because vegetations are often less than 0.2 cm in size
- [ ] C It almost never occurs in people with normal heart valves
- [ ] D Metastatic abscess is seen more commonly in subacute endocarditis than in acute endocarditis
- [ ] E A cardiac conduction defect is often due to associated acute coronary insufficiency

2.8   A 57-year-old woman is admitted with Gram-negative
       septicaemia. She is given intravenous antibiotics and normal
       saline. Two days later, she becomes anxious, tachypnoeic and
       short of breath. An emergency chest X-ray demonstrates diffuse,
       bilateral interstitial and alveolar infiltrates. Her past medical
       history revealed hypertension and that she has been on regular
       antihypertensive treatment for 7 years. She has never had any
       evidence of congestive heart failure. In this case, adult
       respiratory distress syndrome can be distinguished from
       cardiogenic pulmonary oedema by which one of the following
       investigations?

☐   A   Measurement of the central venous pressure
☐   B   Calculation of the alveolar–arterial Po_2 difference
☐   C   Measurement of the pulmonary artery wedge pressure
☐   D   Measurement of lung compliance
☐   E   Measurement of the ejection fraction

2.9   A 30-year-old woman presents with a 3-month history of chest
       pain. On auscultation, there is a mid-systolic click and a late
       systolic murmur. Her ECG shows T-wave inversion in leads II, III
       and aVF. Which one of the following statements concerning her
       condition is true?

☐   A   The patient's chest pain could be due to associated coronary
          artery disease
☐   B   The click and murmur occur earlier in systole when the
          patient stands up
☐   C   An exercise stress test would most likely be positive
☐   D   Asymmetrical hypertrophy of the interventricular septum is
          revealed on echocardiography
☐   E   Prophylactic measures to prevent subacute bacterial
          endocarditis are not warranted

2.10   A 60-year-old man is admitted with shortness of breath. On examination, you hear a musical ejection systolic murmur at the lower sternal edge, radiating to both carotids. The echocardiogram shows a thickened aortic valve and there is a 50-mmHg pressure gradient across the valve. Which one of the following is the most common cause of this valve abnormality?

☐   A   Bicuspid aortic valve disease
☐   B   Left ventricular membrane
☐   C   Hypertrophic obstructive cardiomyopathy (HOCM)
☐   D   Rheumatic fever
☐   E   Cystic medial necrosis

2.11   A 44-year-old man being investigated for non-specific chest pain and shortness of breath is found to have left bundle branch block on a 12-lead ECG. Which one of the following conditions is most likely to be associated with this ECG abnormality?

☐   A   Ischaemic heart disease
☐   B   Mitral stenosis
☐   C   Pericarditis
☐   D   Pulmonary embolism
☐   E   Tricuspid stenosis

2.12   A 68-year-old man is admitted with rapid deterioration in his general health, with fatigue and excessive tiredness. He claims that his health has been in decline for 2 months. He has an ejection systolic murmur and his temperature is 37.9 °C. The blood culture is positive from two bottles for *Streptococcus bovis*. Which one of the following statements is true?

☐   A   *Streptococcus bovis* is part of the normal oral flora
☐   B   Echocardiography would add little to this patient's management
☐   C   Intravenous gentamicin plus amoxicillin is the treatment of choice
☐   D   *Streptococcus bovis* is a Gram-negative coccus
☐   E   Barium enema would be advised to exclude colonic malignancy

2.13   **A pregnant 28-year-old woman is being examined during a routine antenatal visit. Which one of the following haemodynamic changes is regarded as physiological during pregnancy?**

- [ ] A   A 20% reduction in blood volume and cardiac output
- [ ] B   A 10-mmHg drop in diastolic blood pressure towards the end of pregnancy
- [ ] C   Bradycardia with a radial pulse rate between 45 and 55 bpm
- [ ] D   A grade 2/6 diastolic murmur over the mitral area
- [ ] E   Pulsus alternans

2.14   **A 55-year-old businessman attends the Outpatients Department with retrosternal chest pain. The pain radiates to the lower jaw and the left arm. He has had several similar attacks in the last 12 months. Eating a heavy meal sometimes causes indigestion and may precipitate the pain. A 12-lead ECG shows T-wave inversion in lead III. Which one of the following is the most reliable feature of chest pain secondary to ischaemic heart disease?**

- [ ] A   Retrosternal location
- [ ] B   Radiation to the lower jaw
- [ ] C   Associated T-wave inversion in lead III on the 12-lead ECG
- [ ] D   Pain aggravated by heavy meals
- [ ] E   Tenderness on palpating the left second costochondral joint

2.15   **A 30-year-old woman presents with pain in the right calf and right-sided chest pain. There is no swelling or tenderness on examination of the leg. In the evaluation for venous thromboembolism, which one of the following is true of plasma D-dimer testing?**

- [ ] A   It has high sensitivity, so a positive test establishes the diagnosis in most patients
- [ ] B   It is usually negative when pulmonary embolism is confined to subsegmental vessels
- [ ] C   It is only positive in venous thromboembolism
- [ ] D   It can reliably distinguish between a ruptured Baker's cyst and deep venous thrombosis
- [ ] E   It has a high negative predictive value, so a negative result almost completely excludes venous thromboembolism

2.16 A healthy 35-year-old man complains of recurrent episodes of giddiness. He denies having any chest pain, palpitations or breathlessness. He also describes having an attack of unprovoked syncope 2 weeks earlier. His otherwise healthy 26-year-old brother died suddenly in his sleep 2 years ago. Clinical examination is unremarkable. The 12-lead ECG shows ST-segment elevation and T-wave inversion in leads V2 and V3. Serial cardiac enzymes are normal and a coronary angiogram reveals normal coronary arteries. A transthoracic echocardiogram shows normal left ventricular systolic size and function. What is the most likely diagnosis?

☐ A Romano–Ward syndrome
☐ B Acute anterior myocardial infarction
☐ C Hypertrophic cardiomyopathy
☐ D Brugada syndrome
☐ E Wolff–Parkinson–White syndrome

2.17 A 60-year-old man has undergone coronary angiography for the investigation of unstable angina. The next day, while recovering in hospital, he complains of severe pain in his right foot, followed by sudden partial loss of sight in the left eye. On examination, the peripheral pulses in the lower limb are palpable and of good volume. There is gangrene of the lateral two toes on the right foot. Fundoscopy reveals cholesterol emboli in a branch of the central retinal artery in the left eye. Which one of the following is the most probable diagnosis in this case?

☐ A Atheroembolic disease
☐ B Polyarteritis nodosa
☐ C Buerger's disease
☐ D Arterial thromboembolism
☐ E Disseminated intravascular coagulopathy

2.18   A 63-year-old man who is known to have tuberculosis is referred
       with shortness of breath and increasing ankle swelling. On
       examination, a raised jugular venous pulse (JVP) and soft heart
       sounds are noted and he has pitting oedema below the knee.
       There is also an inspiratory increase in venous pressure and a
       steep y descent in the JVP. Which one of the following is the most
       likely diagnosis?

☐   A   Constrictive pericarditis
☐   B   Active pulmonary tuberculosis
☐   C   Cor pulmonale
☐   D   Cardiac tamponade
☐   E   Right-sided heart failure

2.19   A 59-year-old man presents with acute shortness of breath,
       epigastric pain and vomiting. Examination reveals a pulse of
       60 bpm and a blood pressure of 60/30 mmHg. The JVP is
       significantly raised; lung and heart examination is within normal
       limits. Investigation reveals ST elevation in leads II, III and aVF on
       a 12-lead ECG . What is the most likely diagnosis?

☐   A   Perforated peptic ulcer
☐   B   Cardiac tamponade
☐   C   Acute ventricular septal defect-associated acute myocardial
        infarction
☐   D   Right ventricular acute myocardial infarction
☐   E   Acute aortic regurgitation-associated acute myocardial
        infarction

2.20   A 76-year-old woman is attending the hospital for regular review. She is found to have atrial fibrillation at a rate of 77 bpm with no evidence of ischaemic heart disease on a 12-lead ECG. Examination of the heart and lungs is otherwise normal. She denies having any symptoms. Thyroid function tests and an echocardiogram are also within normal limits. The past medical history is unremarkable apart from hypertension, which is well controlled with atenolol 50 mg/day. She tells you that her doctor has told her on several occasions in the past that her heart beats irregularly. Which of the following is the most appropriate action at this stage?

☐   A   No further action and arrange further review in 4 months
☐   B   Start digoxin therapy
☐   C   Start flecainide
☐   D   Warfarin therapy should be initiated to keep the INR between 2 and 3
☐   E   Prescribe amiodarone

Chapter 3

CLINICAL PHARMACOLOGY AND TOXICOLOGY

Questions

3.1 A 76-year-old man has been found by neighbours sitting in his chair with vomitus on his chest. He was semiconscious. They broke into his house when he failed to collect milk bottles left on the doorstep for 4 days. He is known to have peripheral vascular disease. He is admitted to the High Dependency Unit. His rectal temperature is 30.4 °C, the 12-lead ECG shows atrial fibrillation with a ventricular rate of 42 bpm and his blood pressure is 120/70 mmHg. In addition to rewarming therapy, which other immediate measure would you consider most appropriate?

- ☐ A Intravenous hydrocortisone 200 mg
- ☐ B Temporary pacemaker
- ☐ C Intravenous atropine
- ☐ D Intravenous thiamine
- ☐ E Insertion of a nasogastric tube and flecainide therapy

3.2 D-penicillamine is an antidote used as a chelating agent for which one of the following heavy metal poisonings?

- ☐ A Thallium
- ☐ B Copper
- ☐ C Arsenic
- ☐ D Lead
- ☐ E Mercury

3.3   A pregnant 31-year-old woman has been found by her husband in the garage, cyanosed and agitated. Apparently, she left the car engine running while she was clearing the garage. She smokes heavily but has no previous medical problems. She has been rushed to the Emergency Department where it is thought that she has carbon monoxide (CO) poisoning. Which one of the following statements is true?

☐ A   The baseline CO may exceed 15% in smokers, compared with 1–3% in non-smokers

☐ B   The affinity of haemoglobin for oxygen is 200–250 times greater than its affinity for CO

☐ C   The fetus is usually protected from the direct effect of CO because the placental microvasculature acts as barrier

☐ D   Venous blood samples are generally not adequate for measurements of CO in the blood

☐ E   Computed tomography (CT) scan of the brain will identify hypodense periventricular lesions which are characteristic of severe CO poisoning

3.4   A 22-year-old student has collapsed. He was with friends and was upset about his final examination results. They say that he has had a lot to drink and has probably taken an overdose of an unknown substance. On examination, he smells of alcohol and is comatose. His pupils are small but there are no localising signs. The full blood count (FBC), glucose, urea and electrolytes (U&Es), liver function tests (LFTs) and INR are all within normal limits. He is intubated and given naloxone intravenously. He becomes more alert but starts to experience abdominal cramps, nausea and vomiting. Which one of the following statements is correct?

☐ A   Naloxone has no pharmacological effect on the central nervous system (CNS) toxicity of ethanol (alcohol)

☐ B   The patient is unlikely to be an opioid addict

☐ C   The plasma paracetamol concentration should be measured urgently

☐ D   Naloxone reverses the effect of all opioids

☐ E   Naloxone is readily deactivated when introduced down the endotracheal tube in an unconscious patient

3.5 Which one of the following antimicrobial drugs has virtually no effect against anaerobic bacteria?

- [ ] A Clindamycin
- [ ] B Amoxicillin
- [ ] C Gentamicin
- [ ] D Tetracycline
- [ ] E Chloramphenicol

3.6 Which one of the following statements about warfarin is most accurate?

- [ ] A It reduces protein C levels in the blood
- [ ] B It may induce autoimmune thrombocytopenia
- [ ] C Chronic use is often associated with osteoporosis
- [ ] D An initial loading dose is given because it has a short half-life (3 hours)
- [ ] E It should be avoided in lactating women

3.7 Which one of the following statements about vancomycin is true?

- [ ] A It inhibits bacterial DNA replication
- [ ] B It has no significant effect on Gram-negative cocci
- [ ] C It is well absorbed when given by mouth, with 90% bioavailability
- [ ] D It is eliminated mainly by liver oxidation
- [ ] E Cardiotoxicity is the main side-effect

3.8 Which one of the following diuretics produces a picture of metabolic acidosis?

- [ ] A Bumetanide
- [ ] B Metolazone
- [ ] C Thiazide diuretics
- [ ] D Furosemide
- [ ] E Acetazolamide

Answers on pages 157–159

3.9   Sulphonylurea therapy is associated with which one of the following effects?

☐ A   It reduces absorption of carbohydrates from the gut
☐ B   It stimulates the pancreas to release stored insulin
☐ C   It reduces hepatic gluconeogenesis
☐ D   It rarely causes clinical hypoglycaemia
☐ E   It increases the utilisation of glucose in peripheral tissues

3.10   Which one of the following statements comparing selective serotonin-reuptake inhibitors (SSRIs) with tricyclic antidepressants is true?

☐ A   SSRIs have more sedative effects
☐ B   Weight gain is a recognised side-effect of SSRIs
☐ C   SSRIs have a less profound antimuscarinic effect
☐ D   SSRIs can be used safely in epileptic patients
☐ E   A drug-free period is not necessary when SSRIs are prescribed to replace monoamine oxidase inhibitors (MAOIs)

3.11   A 61-year-old woman with progressive, unexplained weight loss and exophthalmos was diagnosed with Graves' disease. She developed an extensive skin reaction to carbimazole. Her doctor is suggesting radioactive iodine as an alternative therapy. Which one of the following statements best describes the use of radioactive iodine (^{131}I) in the treatment of thyrotoxicosis?

☐ A   Triple-dose therapy (1 month apart) is the standard regime used in most cases
☐ B   It is given by intravenous infusion to avoid gastrointestinal toxicity
☐ C   It is not associated with an increased incidence of late leukaemia
☐ D   Hypoparathyroidism secondary to β emissions and ablation of the parathyroid gland occurs in 30% of cases
☐ E   Rapid regression of exophthalmos is expected in almost all cases within the first 3 months

3.12 Which one of the following statements about drug-induced liver disease is accurate?

☐ A Isoniazid typically causes liver damage in slow acetylators
☐ B Halothane hepatitis usually becomes evident approximately 7–10 days after anaesthesia
☐ C Erythromycin stearate can cause cholestasis
☐ D Flucloxacillin therapy characteristically causes liver granuloma
☐ E Chronic use of aspirin in excess of 3 g/day causes hepatoma

3.13 Which one of the following antiplatelet agents acts by inhibiting the phosphodiesterase enzyme and increasing the cellular concentration of cyclic adenosine monophosphate (cAMP)?

☐ A Abciximab
☐ B Ticlopidine
☐ C Aspirin
☐ D Clopidogrel
☐ E Dipyridamole

3.14 Beta-blockers (β-adrenergic agents) are used in the treatment of angina because they have which one of the following properties?

☐ A They increase sinus node automaticity
☐ B They increase the left atrial volume and pressure
☐ C They increase the peripheral vascular resistance
☐ D They decrease the heart rate and myocardial contractility
☐ E They increase the preload

3.15 An obese 40-year-old teacher is determined to lose weight. She exercises three times a week at the local gym and is on a slimming diet. Last month she managed to lose 3 kg in weight and is now asking your opinion about initiating orlistat therapy. On advising her, you would explain that orlistat therapy has which one of the following effects?

☐ A It prevents fat absorption from the intestine
☐ B It improves the bone mineral density
☐ C It causes dramatic weight loss in the first month
☐ D It increases the cholesterol level in the first year of therapy
☐ E It increases the risk of clotting

Answers on pages 159–162

3.16   Propylthiouracil has a modest therapeutic advantage over carbimazole in the treatment of thyrotoxicosis because it has which one of the following properties?

☐   A   It inhibits the organification of iodine in the thyroid gland
☐   B   It is not excreted in breast milk
☐   C   It is more potent
☐   D   It has a different chemical structure and so does not share the same adverse effects profile
☐   E   It inhibits the conversion of T4 to T3

3.17   Which one of the following cytotoxic agents is associated with cardiotoxicity?

☐   A   Doxorubicin
☐   B   Cyclophosphamide
☐   C   Cisplatin
☐   D   Bleomycin
☐   E   Vincristine

3.18   A 65-year-old woman with type 2 diabetes of 11 years' duration presents with poorly controlled blood glucose levels. She was overweight and was initially started on metformin therapy. Her diabetes was well controlled until the last 12 months. Despite strict adherence to diet, exercise and maximum daily doses of metformin, satisfactory blood glucose control has proved difficult to achieve and the last HbA_{1c} was 13%. You consider adding rosiglitazone. Which one of the following describes this agent?

☐   A   A benzoic acid derivative
☐   B   An α-glucosidase inhibitor
☐   C   An insulin secretagogue which stimulates insulin secretion by the β cells
☐   D   A sulphonylurea
☐   E   An insulin sensitiser which decreases peripheral insulin resistance

3.19 **Which one of the following antihypertensive agents controls the blood pressure by blocking peripheral α_1-adrenoceptors?**

- ☐ A Losartan
- ☐ B Doxazosin
- ☐ C Minoxidil
- ☐ D Methyldopa
- ☐ E Clonidine

3.20 **A 50-year-old man who is known to have angina is referred with increasing chest pain on exertion. He is currently taking aspirin and a β-blocker. You decide to add oral nitrate to his medication. Which one of the following contribute to the beneficial effect of glyceryl trinitrate?**

- ☐ A Reduction of oxygen transport to the myocardium
- ☐ B Dilatation of systemic veins
- ☐ C Increase in left ventricular preload
- ☐ D Reduction in sodium and potassium transport in myocardial muscle
- ☐ E Increase in left ventricular afterload

3.21 **Three months ago, a 67-year-old woman with heart failure was prescribed an angiotensin-converting enzyme (ACE) inhibitor and diuretics. She felt much better but she is now troubled by a persistent dry cough. Which one of the following factors is most probably responsible for causing this cough?**

- ☐ A Increased angiotensin in the circulation
- ☐ B Increased bradykinin concentration
- ☐ C Low potassium levels in the bronchioles
- ☐ D Bronchial dehydration caused by chronic diuretic therapy
- ☐ E Recurrent chest infection

3.22 **Which one of the following is true regarding amiodarone?**

- ☐ A Approximately 5% of its weight is iodine
- ☐ B It causes shortening of the QT interval
- ☐ C It has calcium-channel-blocking properties
- ☐ D It has no effect on potassium channels
- ☐ E It promotes renal excretion of digoxin when used concomitantly

Answers on pages 162–165

3.23 Ximelagatran is one of a group of new oral anticoagulant drugs which is going to be introduced, pending further studies. It is thought that it is likely to become the standard oral therapy for long-term anticoagulation. Which one of the following statements about ximelagatran use is correct?

☐ A It acts by direct inhibition of thrombin
☐ B It is metabolised by the hepatic cytochrome P450 system
☐ C Physicians will have to avoid the same drugs that interact with warfarin
☐ D The INR should be used to monitor ximelagatran dosage
☐ E Parenteral vitamin K is a direct antidote, which helps to control serious bleeding complicating ximelagatran use

3.24 A middle-aged diabetic man has been diagnosed with erectile dysfunction and he has asked if he could be prescribed sildenafil (Viagra®). He is on a number of other drugs. You believe that sildenafil is contraindicated because he regularly uses which one of the following medications?

☐ A Rosiglitazone
☐ B Aspirin
☐ C Sublingual glyceryl trinitrate
☐ D ACE inhibitor
☐ E Metformin

3.25 With respect to the intrapulmonary delivery of insulin (ie inhaled), which one of the following statements is true?

☐ A Cigarette smoking has no effect on absorption of inhaled insulin
☐ B It abolishes the need for subcutaneous insulin injections in type 1 diabetes
☐ C 10–30% of the inhaled dose of insulin is absorbed into the circulation
☐ D When used alone, it offers adequate glycaemic control for patients with type 1 diabetes
☐ E It results in a deterioration in pulmonary function

3.26 **Which one of the following pharmacokinetic parameters remains normal in chronic renal failure?**

☐ A Absorption
☐ B Protein binding
☐ C Volume of distribution
☐ D Renal metabolism of drugs
☐ E Bioavailability immediately following intravenous injection of a drug

3.27 **In renal drug elimination, the extraction ratio can be defined as which one of the following?**

☐ A The decline of drug concentration in the plasma from the arterial to the venous side of the kidney
☐ B A measure of the time during which the concentration of the drug in the plasma falls by 50%
☐ C The proportion of an orally administered drug which reaches the circulation
☐ D The ratio of drug concentration in the urine to drug concentration in the bile
☐ E The concentration of a drug in the urine divided by the concentration in the plasma

3.28 **A 66-year-old man is referred for urgent assessment. A routine preoperative blood test shows his potassium level to be 6.6 mmol/l. Which one of the following disorders could be responsible for this abnormality?**

☐ A Bartter's syndrome
☐ B Treatment with corticosteroids
☐ C Liquorice addiction
☐ D Liddle's syndrome
☐ E Ciclosporin therapy

3.29   A 53-year-old man is referred to the Emergency Department with deterioration in level of consciousness and convulsions. He is known to suffer with bipolar depression and is taking lithium on a regular basis. The lithium level is 4.3 mmol/l. Which one of the following is the most appropriate treatment?

☐   A   Activated charcoal
☐   B   Methionine
☐   C   Haemodialysis
☐   D   Forced diuresis with sodium chloride
☐   E   Methylprednisolone

3.30   In relation to acute interstitial nephritis, which one of the following statements is correct?

☐   A   Bilaterally small kidneys is a typical finding on ultrasound scan
☐   B   The condition is caused by direct tubular toxicity
☐   C   Allopurinol is a known cause
☐   D   Haematuria is typically absent
☐   E   Impaired renal function is not a feature in uncomplicated cases

3.31   Which one of the following features is most characteristic of lead poisoning?

☐   A   A predominantly sensory peripheral neuropathy
☐   B   Posterior uveitis
☐   C   Punctate basophilic stippling on peripheral blood film examination
☐   D   Membranous glomerulonephritis as the primary kidney lesion
☐   E   A gingival blue line in children

Answers on pages 168–170

Chapter 4

DERMATOLOGY

Questions

4.1 A 61-year-old man presents with a 1-week history of cough and haemoptysis. The chest X-ray shows dense consolidation in the right lower lobe. Examination of the skin shows concentric erythematous bands forming a woodgrain appearance on the trunk and upper arm. Which one of the following diagnoses is most consistent with this skin rash?

- ☐ A Erythema marginatum
- ☐ B Erythema gyratum repens
- ☐ C Erythema chronicum migrans
- ☐ D Erythema multiforme
- ☐ E Erythema nodosum

4.2 Which one of the following conditions is most likely to be associated with pyoderma gangrenosum?

- ☐ A Tuberculosis
- ☐ B Leprosy
- ☐ C Chronic myeloid leukaemia
- ☐ D Sulphonamide therapy
- ☐ E Cushing's syndrome

4.3 Vitiligo is associated with which one of the following disorders?

- ☐ A Nelson's syndrome
- ☐ B Hyperparathyroidism
- ☐ C Amiodarone therapy
- ☐ D Addison's disease
- ☐ E Chronic renal failure

4.4   **Which one of the following disorders is most commonly associated with Stevens–Johnson syndrome?**

- [ ] A   Herpes simplex infection
- [ ] B   Sarcoidosis
- [ ] C   Systemic lupus erythematosus
- [ ] D   Herpes zoster infection
- [ ] E   Coeliac disease

4.5   **Which one of the following is known to be associated with photosensitivity?**

- [ ] A   Statin therapy
- [ ] B   Rheumatoid arthritis
- [ ] C   Hyperthyroidism
- [ ] D   Scurvy
- [ ] E   Porphyria cutanea tarda

4.6   **The Koebner phenomenon is encountered in which one of the following conditions?**

- [ ] A   Lupus vulgaris
- [ ] B   Pityriasis rosea
- [ ] C   Psoriasis
- [ ] D   Erythema nodosum
- [ ] E   Squamous-cell carcinoma of the skin

4.7   **A 23-year-old homosexual man visits a local doctor while on holiday in the UK from Australia. He has noted a lesion on his penis that was initially nodular and painless, but which has progressed over time to form a heaped-up ulcer. Sampling from the lesion reveals large infected mononuclear cells containing many Donovan bodies. Which one of the following diagnoses fits best with this clinical picture?**

- [ ] A   Penile carcinoma
- [ ] B   Lymphogranuloma venereum
- [ ] C   Chancroid
- [ ] D   Genital herpes
- [ ] E   Granuloma inguinale

4.8 A 24-year-old woman with type 1 diabetes attends your clinic for review. She presents with small, intensely itchy blisters on her skin. These are present particularly on her elbows, extensor aspects of her forearms, scalp and buttocks. Some of the blisters have been de-roofed and present as erosions. She has been treated in the past for chronic diarrhoea, presumed to be due to diabetic neuropathy. Which one of the diagnoses below fits best with this clinical picture?

- ☐ A Folliculitis related to diabetes
- ☐ B Eczema
- ☐ C Dermatitis herpetiformis
- ☐ D Linear IgA disease
- ☐ E Epidermolysis bullosa

4.9 A 25-year-old man presents with a well-defined patch of hair loss on his scalp surrounded by 'exclamation mark' broken hairs. He also has nail pitting and hypopigmented skin, but no scarring. Which one of the following is the most likely diagnosis?

- ☐ A Alopecia areata
- ☐ B Discoid lupus
- ☐ C Telogen effluvium
- ☐ D Trichotillomania
- ☐ E Tinea capitis

4.10 A 20-year-old woman with acne vulgaris has been started on isotretinoin. Which one of the following statements about treatment with isotretinoin is accurate?

- ☐ A It is contraindicated in patients with renal artery stenosis
- ☐ B It can cause hirsutism
- ☐ C It can cause hyperkalaemia and electrolytes should be checked every month
- ☐ D Pregnancy should be avoided during and for 1 month after treatment
- ☐ E It may cause haemoptysis

Chapter 5

ENDOCRINOLOGY AND METABOLIC DISORDERS

Questions

5.1 You have received a blood test report with the following results: serum calcium 3 mmol/l, serum phosphate 0.6 mmol/l (normal range 0.8–1.4 mmol/l); plasma parathyroid hormone (PTH) 5.8 pmol/l (normal range 0.9–5.4 pmol/l). Which one of the following disorders could be associated with this abnormal blood test?

- [ ] A   Addison's disease
- [ ] B   DiGeorge syndrome
- [ ] C   Mucocutaneous candidiasis
- [ ] D   Medullary-cell carcinoma
- [ ] E   Magnesium deficiency

5.2 In a patient with persistent hypokalaemia, the presence of a normal blood pressure after prolonged periods of follow-up would be most suggestive of which one of the following disorders?

- [ ] A   Renal artery stenosis
- [ ] B   Liddle's syndrome
- [ ] C   Conn's syndrome
- [ ] D   Cushing's syndrome
- [ ] E   Bartter's syndrome

5.3   The blood gas analysis in a 40-year-old woman who has presented
       with fatigue shows: pH 7.51, PaO_2 11 kPa, $PaCO_2$ 6 kPa,
       bicarbonate 32 mmol/l. Which one of the following is the most
       likely cause of this patient's clinical presentation?

☐   A   Spironolactone therapy
☐   B   Acetazolamide therapy
☐   C   Conn's syndrome
☐   D   Addison's disease
☐   E   Chronic diarrhoea

5.4   A 33-year-old woman presents with breast congestion. She says
       that milk is expressed freely from the nipples every time she
       squeezes her breast. She takes two drugs but she does not know
       their names. Which one of the following disorders could explain
       this patient's presentation?

☐   A   Turner's syndrome
☐   B   Polycystic ovary disease
☐   C   Myxoedema
☐   D   Sheehan's syndrome
☐   E   Bromocriptine therapy

5.5   A 40-year-old woman presents with sinus tachycardia and
       proximal muscle weakness. She is found to have a free T4 of
       33 pmol/l (normal range 10–24 pmol/l) and a TSH of 0.001 mU/l
       (normal range 0.3–4.0 mU/l). Which one of the following
       features is associated with this disorder?

☐   A   Menorrhagia
☐   B   Excessive hair loss
☐   C   Weight gain
☐   D   Pretibial myxoedema
☐   E   Peripheral neuropathy

5.6   A 49-year-old man with medullary thyroid cancer was found to
       have a serum total calcium concentration of 3.4 mmol/l and a
       phosphate of 0.57 mmol/l on preoperative blood testing. Intact
       parathyroid hormone (PTH) was 38.0 pmol/l (normal range
       0.9–5.4 pmol/l). Primary hyperparathyroidism was diagnosed.
       Examination reveals the patient to have a short systolic murmur
       and a blood pressure of 180/100 mmHg. Which of the following
       is the most appropriate test to organise at this stage?

☐   A   24-hour urine catecholamines
☐   B   Gastrin
☐   C   Prolactin
☐   D   Serum protein electrophoresis
☐   E   Serum angiotensin-converting enzyme

5.7   A pregnant 28-year-old woman is referred for investigation of
       tachycardia and weight loss. She is found to have
       hyperthyroidism and exophthalmos. Which one of the following
       statements about this condition is true?

☐   A   Neonatal hyperthyroidism is unlikely if the maternal thyroxine
            level is strictly controlled during pregnancy
☐   B   Carbimazole is absolutely contraindicated
☐   C   Surgery can be performed safely in the second trimester
☐   D   The presence of persistent exophthalmos indicates poor
            control of the active disease
☐   E   Antithyroid drugs do not enter breast milk

5.8   An 18-year-old man is admitted with deep-sighing respiration and
       irritability. His friend says that he has been vomiting. Urgent
       blood gas analysis shows the following: pH 7.26, bicarbonate
       17 mmol/l, PaO_2 14 kPa, $PaCO_2$ 3.4 kPa. The serum sodium is
       140 mmol/l, potassium 5.5 mmol/l and chloride 98 mmol/l. The
       renal function reveals: creatinine 140 μmol/l, urea 8 mmol/l.
       Which of the following is the most likely cause of this patient's
       acute deterioration?

☐   A   Acetazolamide therapy
☐   B   Renal tubular acidosis type 2
☐   C   Hyperventilation
☐   D   Aspirin overdose
☐   E   Persistent vomiting

5.9   A pregnant 23-year-old woman was found to have a fasting blood glucose in the region of 8–9 mmol/l on several antenatal checks. Blood glucose levels just before her pregnancy were normal. In this situation, which one of the following statements is true?

☐   A   The hyperglycaemia is mild and diet control is all that is required
☐   B   50% will go on to develop maturity-onset diabetes mellitus
☐   C   This has no tendency to recur in subsequent pregnancies
☐   D   Unlike pregnant diabetics, there is no increase in the risk of fetal macrosomia in this patient
☐   E   The risk of congenital malformation is increased

5.10   A 60-year-old chronic alcoholic is admitted with delirium tremens and is found to have a serum phosphate of 0.2 mmol/l (normal range 0.8–1.4 mmol/l). This might lead to which one of the following possible complications?

☐   A   Carpopedal spasm
☐   B   Rhabdomyolysis
☐   C   Cardiac arrythmia
☐   D   Metastatic calcification
☐   E   Constipation

5.11   Which one of the following proteins is most likely to be associated with very high levels of plasma chylomicrons?

☐   A   Apoprotein E
☐   B   Apoprotein C-II
☐   C   Apoprotein A-II
☐   D   Lipoprotein B
☐   E   LDL (low-density lipoprotein) receptor

5.12 A 65-year-old woman with chronic low back pain develops a severe sharp pain in the left groin after a minor fall and is unable to walk. A left neck of femur fracture is identified on radiological examination. Routine laboratory evaluation discloses a low serum calcium concentration of 1.9 mmol/l, a serum phosphate concentration of 0.78 mmol/l and increased serum alkaline phosphatase activity. The serum parathyroid hormone level is subsequently found to be elevated. Which of the following is the most likely diagnosis?

- [ ] A Primary hyperparathyroidism
- [ ] B Hypervitaminosis D
- [ ] C Paget's disease of bone
- [ ] D Osteoporosis
- [ ] E Vitamin D deficiency

5.13 A 45-year-old woman presents with general weakness and unexplained fatigue. Investigation reveals a serum potassium concentration of 2.2 mmol/l. Which of the following is the most likely diagnosis?

- [ ] A Metabolic acidosis
- [ ] B Renal tubular acidosis
- [ ] C Spironolactone therapy
- [ ] D Addison's disease
- [ ] E Haemolytic anaemia

5.14 Eight days ago, a 67-year-old man was referred to the Emergency Department with a serum calcium of 3.2 mmol/l. He was admitted to hospital and a trial of prednisolone 30 mg daily was started. There has been no change in his condition and the serum calcium is now 3.3 mmol/l. This patient's hypercalcaemia is most likely to be due to which one of the following conditions?

- [ ] A Sarcoidosis
- [ ] B Primary hyperparathyroidism
- [ ] C Hypervitaminosis D
- [ ] D Multiple myeloma
- [ ] E Malignancy with bone metastases

5.15   A 33-year-old man is referred for the management of hyperlipidaemia. He is found to have palmar xanthomata. What is the most likely cause of hyperlipidaemia in this patient?

- [ ] A   Familial hypercholesterolaemia
- [ ] B   Familial hypertriglyceridaemia
- [ ] C   Familial dysbetalipoproteinaemia
- [ ] D   Familial combined hyperlipidaemia
- [ ] E   Lipoprotein lipase deficiency

5.16   Which one of the following clinical features is characteristic of insulin resistance?

- [ ] A   Acanthosis nigricans
- [ ] B   Nephropathy
- [ ] C   Retinopathy
- [ ] D   Peripheral neuropathy
- [ ] E   Hypoglycaemia

5.17   A 66-year-old man has been diagnosed with glucagonoma. He presented with a skin lesion covering the left side of his face. Which of the following is the most likely diagnosis of this skin lesion?

- [ ] A   Erythema chronicum migrans
- [ ] B   Acanthosis nigricans
- [ ] C   Panniculitis
- [ ] D   Ichthyosis
- [ ] E   Necrolytic migratory erythema

5.18   A 56-year-old woman who is known to have hypothyroidism and who is currently taking thyroxine at a dose of 100 µg/day is admitted to the Orthopaedic Unit with a left hip fracture after a fall at home. A bone mineral density (BMD) assessment of the opposite femur confirms the diagnosis of osteoporosis, with a T-score of –2.8. She is prescribed alendronate 70 mg weekly. Which one of the following statements is true?

☐   A   Excessive thyroxine is an additional risk factor for osteoporosis
☐   B   Plain X-rays of bone are sensitive enough to identify low BMD
☐   C   The T-score compares a patient's BMD with the mean value for people of the same age and sex
☐   D   A high serum phosphate level may be suggestive of hyperparathyroidism
☐   E   Bisphosphonates such as alendronate act by inhibiting bone formation

5.19   Hypogonadism in boys is a feature of which one of the following disorders?

☐   A   Primary hypothyroidism
☐   B   Craniopharyngioma
☐   C   Tuberous sclerosis
☐   D   Hepatoblastoma
☐   E   Gigantism

5.20   Which one of the following statements is true with regard to dietary deficiency?

☐   A   Zinc deficiency causes acrodermatitis and altered taste
☐   B   Manganese deficiency is associated with peptic ulcer disease
☐   C   Haemolytic anaemia may result from chromium deficiency
☐   D   Copper deficiency causes Wilson's disease
☐   E   Selenium deficiency causes peripheral neuropathy

5.21   **Which one of the following statements is true with regard to postpartum thyroiditis?**

- [ ] A   It typically occurs in the first week after delivery
- [ ] B   Hyperthyroidism predominates in the clinical picture during the course of this condition
- [ ] C   Spontaneous recovery is expected in 90% of cases
- [ ] D   Positive antimicrosomal antibodies help to differentiate it from Graves' disease
- [ ] E   Radioactive iodine uptake is usually intense

5.22   **Blood levels of high-density lipoproteins are increased by which one of the following?**

- [ ] A   Aspirin therapy
- [ ] B   Alcohol ingestion
- [ ] C   Angiotensin-converting enzyme (ACE) inhibitor therapy
- [ ] D   Treatment with β-blockers
- [ ] E   Diabetes mellitus

5.23   **A 50-year-old woman with type 2 diabetes treated with glibenclamide was admitted because of recurrent blackouts. Investigations show impaired renal function, with a serum creatinine of 233 µmol/l. Two hours after admission, her level of consciousness decreased and she became unresponsive to physical stimuli. Her blood glucose was found to be 1.1 mmol/l and she was treated with an intravenous bolus of 50 ml of 50% glucose, which promptly restored consciousness. A continuous intravenous infusion of 5% glucose was started and her blood glucose concentration was measured 2-hourly throughout the night. The glibenclamide was discontinued. Next morning, what would the most appropriate course of action be?**

- [ ] A   Keep her nil-by-mouth and continue with intravenous 5% glucose for at least 48 hours
- [ ] B   Try subcutaneous glucagon to prevent further hypoglycaemic episodes
- [ ] C   Discharge home, because further episodes are unlikely as the oral hypoglycaemic drug was stopped
- [ ] D   Try octreotide to control further hypoglycaemic attacks
- [ ] E   Replace the oral hypoglycaemic drug with long-acting insulin if the blood glucose is stable

5.24 A 42-year-old man with long-standing HIV infection presents for review. He has been taking antiretroviral therapy for 5 years and has been relatively free of associated disease. You notice on examination that he appears to have lost subcutaneous fat on his arms, legs and face, and has increased deposition of fat around his abdomen. His lipids are also abnormal, with a raised triglyceride level and low HDL cholesterol. What is the most likely cause of this clinical picture?

A   Antiretroviral-related lipodystrophy
B   HIV wasting
C   HIV-associated malignancy
D   Underlying gastrointestinal pathology
E   An inherited insulin-resistance syndrome

5.25 A 42-year-old man is referred to the Hypertension Clinic for advice. He is currently taking atenolol, bendroflumethiazide and ramipril and his blood pressure is 165/105 mmHg. His serum potassium is 3.0 mmol/l, with a serum bicarbonate of 28 mmol/l. What is the best next management step?

A   Measure the aldosterone : renin ratio
B   Wash out as many of his antihypertensive agents as possible for a period of 2 weeks, then review
C   Take a 24-hour blood pressure recording
D   Arrange 24-hour urinary free-cortisol collection
E   Add in a further agent and review in 12 months

Chapter 6

GASTROENTEROLOGY

Questions

6.1 You are called to see a group of holidaymakers who have developed diarrhoea and abdominal pain. They arrived a week ago at an aqua holiday camp. Stool smear examination shows oocysts when treated with a modified acid-fast stain. What is the most likely diagnosis?

- A   Giardiasis
- B   Amoebic dysentery
- C   Tuberculous enteritis
- D   Cryptosporidiosis
- E   Staphylococcal food poisoning

6.2 A 32-year-old woman presents with diarrhoea, with mucus and blood in the stool, and recurrent abdominal pain. Colonoscopy is performed and a mucosal biopsy is obtained. Which one of the following pathological findings would make ulcerative colitis a more likely diagnosis than Crohn's disease?

- A   Ileal involvement
- B   Crypt abscesses
- C   Transmural involvement
- D   Granulomas
- E   Skip lesions

6.3 **A 45-year-old man is being investigated for persistent dyspepsia and heartburn. Acid secretion studies show gastric acid hypersecretion. Which one of the following conditions is the most likely cause of this patient's symptoms?**

- [ ] A   Pernicious anaemia
- [ ] B   Large-bowel resection
- [ ] C   Vasoactive intestinal polypeptide- (VIP-) secreting tumour
- [ ] D   Systemic mastocytosis
- [ ] E   Cushing's syndrome

6.4 **A 50-year-old woman is admitted with acute diarrhoea and dehydration. Just prior to her admission, she had a bout of lower urinary tract infection and is on antibiotics. Stool culture is negative and sigmoidoscopy reveals pseudomembranous colitis. Which one of the following statements is most characteristic of this patient's condition?**

- [ ] A   Bloody diarrhoea, abdominal pain and tenderness is the most common presentation
- [ ] B   The detection of *Clostridium difficile* bacilli in the stool is diagnostic
- [ ] C   A severe form of the disease is often associated with gentamicin therapy
- [ ] D   It is caused by a Gram-positive anaerobic bacterium
- [ ] E   Intravenous vancomycin for 2 weeks is an effective treatment

6.5 **A 40-year-old woman presents with a 6-month history of chronic diarrhoea and a 6-kg weight loss. Jejunal biopsy findings could provide a definitive diagnosis in which one of the following conditions?**

- [ ] A   Coeliac disease
- [ ] B   Blind loop syndrome
- [ ] C   Tropical sprue
- [ ] D   Intestinal lymphoma
- [ ] E   Giardiasis

6.6   A 33-year-old woman with long-standing ulcerative colitis presents with intestinal obstruction. Colonoscopy shows a constricting lesion in the colon. Biopsy specimens confirm adenocarcinoma of the colon. Which one of the following statements regarding adenocarcinoma of the colon complicating ulcerative colitis is correct?

☐   A   Carcinoembryonic antigen (CEA) is a reliable screening test
☐   B   The risk of carcinoma is higher if the colitis is confined to the left-sided colon
☐   C   Mucosal dysplasia on colon biopsy is associated with the likelihood of carcinoma elsewhere in the bowel
☐   D   The ulcerative colitis is often confined to the last 15 cm of the sigmoid colon
☐   E   The prognosis is more favourable than that of colonic adenocarcinoma developing in the absence of colitis

6.7   A 27-year-old woman presents with a 12-month history of general fatigue and jaundice. She has also noticed an acneiform eruption covering her face and upper chest. The liver function tests show: bilirubin 90 μmol/l, ALT 755 U/l, INR 1.5 and albumin 29 g/l. She is antinuclear antibody- (ANA-) positive and the IgG is raised. What is the most likely diagnosis?

☐   A   Autoimmune hepatitis
☐   B   Primary biliary cirrhosis
☐   C   Alcoholic liver disease
☐   D   Sclerosing cholangitis
☐   E   Gilbert's syndrome

6.8   A 60-year-old man presents with a spiking fever and right hypochondrial pain. Examination reveals an enlarged, tender liver. Which one of the following features would be most suggestive of amoebic liver abscess?

☐   A   Patient usually aged over 60
☐   B   Recent bowel surgery
☐   C   Raised white cell count
☐   D   History of recent biliary colic and fever
☐   E   Solitary abscess in the right lobe of the liver

6.9   A 28-year-old woman is referred for further investigation of weight loss and increasing pallor. Physical examination and abdominal ultrasound are within normal limits. Blood tests show: haemoglobin 8.9 g/dl, MCV 88 fl; serum ferritin 3 µg/l (normal range 15–300 µg/l), serum folate 0.5 µg/l (normal range 2.0–11.0 µg/l); and a normal B12 level. What is the most appropriate test to perform to reach a diagnosis in this patient?

- [ ]   A   Antimitochondrial antibodies
- [ ]   B   Antinuclear antibodies
- [ ]   C   Carcinoembryonic antigen (CEA)
- [ ]   D   Anti-endomyseal antibodies
- [ ]   E   Antiparietal cell antibodies

6.10   Which one of the following statements about carcinoid tumour is true?

- [ ]   A   It is most commonly found in the ileum
- [ ]   B   Carcinoid syndrome can manifest in the absence of liver metastases
- [ ]   C   Aortic stenosis is the most common heart valve abnormality in advanced carcinoid tumour
- [ ]   D   Carcinoid flush is often associated with an instant rise in diastolic blood pressure
- [ ]   E   Banana ingestion can block the renal clearance of 5-hydroxyindoleacetic acid (5-HIAA) and result in false-negative test results

6.11   A 30-year-old man presents with rapidly accumulating ascites and an enlarged liver. Ultrasound of the liver shows a mass in the right lobe of the liver. Liver biopsy confirms the diagnosis of hepatocellular carcinoma. Which one of the following conditions is associated with an increased incidence of this carcinoma?

- [ ]   A   Crigler–Najjar syndrome
- [ ]   B   *Plamodium falciparum* malaria
- [ ]   C   Homozygous α_1-antitrypsin deficiency
- [ ]   D   Wilson's disease
- [ ]   E   Cystic fibrosis

6.12   A 60-year-old male civil servant who has rheumatoid arthritis and
        is taking naproxen 500 mg/day is found to have three duodenal
        ulcers and a 2-cm antral ulcer on upper gastrointestinal
        endoscopy. Abdominal computed tomography shows a 4-cm
        mass in the head of the pancreas. What is the most probable
        diagnosis?

        ☐   A   *Helicobacter pylori*-induced multiple peptic ulcers
        ☐   B   Pancreatic lymphoma
        ☐   C   Glucagonoma
        ☐   D   NSAID-induced upper gastrointestinal ulcers
        ☐   E   Gastrinoma

6.13   A 40-year-old man presents with severe upper abdominal pain
        and vomiting. The serum amylase is very high and a diagnosis of
        acute pancreatitis is confirmed. Which of the following
        conditions is the most likely cause of this patient's pancreatitis?

        ☐   A   Rheumatoid arthritis
        ☐   B   Irritable bowel syndrome
        ☐   C   Hyperlipidaemia
        ☐   D   Hypoparathyroidism
        ☐   E   Diabetes mellitus

6.14   A 50-year-old man presents with recurrent attacks of severe
        epigastric pain that usually radiates to his back. A plain X-ray of
        his abdomen shows small areas of punctate calcification in the
        pancreas. Which one of the following statements is true?

        ☐   A   This patient almost certainly suffers from chronic pancreatitis
        ☐   B   Pancreatic calcification is often an incidental finding and
                carries no clinical significance
        ☐   C   Computed tomography (CT) of the abdomen is mandatory at
                this stage to exclude pancreatic adenocarcinoma with
                calcification
        ☐   D   This is usually the result of passing common bile duct stones
        ☐   E   Pancreatic biopsy would be useful to reach a definitive
                diagnosis

6.15   An obese 55-year-old woman complains of nausea, bloating and reduced exercise tolerance. An abdominal ultrasound shows fatty liver but no other abnormalities. Which one of the following conditions could explain this ultrasound abnormality?

- ☐   A   Obesity
- ☐   B   Primary biliary cirrhosis
- ☐   C   Congestive cardiac failure
- ☐   D   Hypercholesterolaemia
- ☐   E   Addison's disease

6.16   A 59-year-old man presents with a recent history of pallor and general fatigue and tiredness. His haemoglobin is 8.3 g/dl, his MCV is 66 fl and the faecal occult blood test is positive; oesophagogastroduodenoscopy shows no abnormalities. In an attempt to identify the cause of this patient's anaemia, which one of the following investigations is the next appropriate investigation?

- ☐   A   Barium swallow
- ☐   B   CT scan of the abdomen
- ☐   C   Angiography
- ☐   D   Colonoscopy
- ☐   E   Small-bowel barium enema

6.17   A pregnant 20-year-old woman is referred for further investigation. She has noticed yellow discoloration of the sclera and dark-coloured urine and has suffered from excessive itching. Which one of the following statements best describes liver diseases during pregnancy?

- ☐   A   Viral hepatitis runs a milder course
- ☐   B   Acute fatty liver of pregnancy correlates with alcohol consumption prior to pregnancy
- ☐   C   An asymptomatic rise in the serum alkaline phosphatase level warrants further investigations to exclude primary biliary cirrhosis
- ☐   D   Cholestasis of pregnancy may recur in a subsequent pregnancy
- ☐   E   There is no evidence that hepatitis B virus can be transmitted vertically to the fetus

6.18   A 63-year-old man presents with fullness behind both ears. Bilateral enlargement of the parotid glands is diagnosed. Which one of the following is the most likely diagnosis?

☐   A   Hypercholesterolaemia
☐   B   Addison's disease
☐   C   Primary hypothyroidism
☐   D   Coeliac disease
☐   E   Sjögren's syndrome

6.19   A 55-year-old man with compensated liver cirrhosis presents to the Emergency Department with agitation and a rapid decline in the level of consciousness. On examination, he is jaundiced and has a flapping tremor. Which one of the following conditions is probably responsible for this patient's deterioration?

☐   A   Fresh bleeding per rectum
☐   B   Hyperkalaemia
☐   C   Acute diarrhoea
☐   D   Diuretic therapy
☐   E   High carbohydrate diet

6.20   Which one of the following disorders is most likely to be associated with *Helicobacter pylori* infection?
☐   A   Non-ulcer dyspepsia
☐   B   Reflux oesophagitis
☐   C   Coeliac disease
☐   D   Gastric lymphoma
☐   E   Achalasia of the cardia

6.21   A heavy, alcoholic, 40-year-old man presents with jaundice and tremor. Laboratory investigations show: serum total bilirubin 87 µmol/l (normal range 1–22 µmol/l), AST 431 U/l (normal range 1–31 U/l), ALT 254 U/l (normal range 5–35 U/l), GGT 474 U/l (normal range 4–35 U/l) and alkaline phosphatase 171 U/l (normal range 45–105 U/l). Which one of the following statements is accurate with regard to alcoholic liver disease?

- [ ] A   Men are more susceptible than women
- [ ] B   In alcoholic hepatitis the AST : ALT ratio is 2 : 1
- [ ] C   Hepatic iron overload is indicative of concomitant heterozygote haemochromatosis
- [ ] D   Alcoholic fatty infiltration is irreversible once established
- [ ] E   Unlike other causes of liver cirrhosis, alcoholic cirrhosis does not progress to hepatoma

6.22   A 44-year-old woman with primary Sjögren's syndrome presents with fatigue and itching. Laboratory investigations show: serum AST 99 U/l, ALT 154 U/l, GGT 474 U/l, and alkaline phosphatase 771 U/l. Serum IgM levels are elevated. Liver biopsy shows bile-duct destruction with a mononuclear cell infiltration. What is the most likely diagnosis?

- [ ] A   Autoimmune hepatitis (lupoid)
- [ ] B   Sclerosing cholangitis
- [ ] C   Cryptogenic liver cirrhosis
- [ ] D   Primary biliary cirrhosis
- [ ] E   Alcoholic liver disease

6.23   A 67-year-old man presents with recent history of altered bowel habit. Blood tests show his haemoglobin to be 8.7 g/dl, with an MCV of 65 fl. Further investigations confirm the diagnosis of bowel cancer. A history of which one of the following conditions would have predisposed this patient to develop colorectal cancer?

- [ ] A   Amoebic dysentery
- [ ] B   Schistosomiasis
- [ ] C   Ureterosigmoid anastomosis
- [ ] D   Intestinal tuberculosis
- [ ] E   Chronic constipation

6.24 A 34-year-old woman is referred for further assessment of progressive weight loss. The patient is thought to have a malabsorption syndrome. Which one of the following conditions would you expect to be associated with a normal urinary D-xylose test?

- ☐ A Coeliac disease
- ☐ B Chronic pancreatitis
- ☐ C Blind loop syndrome
- ☐ D Chronic renal failure
- ☐ E Liver cirrhosis with ascites

6.25 A middle-aged man presents with haematemesis and melaena. Examination reveals jaundice, spider naevi and gynaecomastia. Ascites and a nodular liver are identified on ultrasound. Which one of the features listed below is a manifestation of portal hypertension?

- ☐ A Jaundice
- ☐ B Gynaecomastia
- ☐ C Spider telangiectases
- ☐ D Hepatomegaly
- ☐ E Oesophageal varices

Chapter 7

GENETICS

Questions

7.1   Which one of the following is most characteristic of achondroplasia?

☐   A   One parent is affected in most cases
☐   B   Absence of osteoclasts in the bone marrow is the hallmark of this disorder
☐   C   The limbs are short but the trunk height is normal
☐   D   Affected individuals are usually sterile
☐   E   Intelligence is subnormal

7.2   Which one of the following is most characteristic of Klinefelter's syndrome?

☐   A   47,XXY karyotype
☐   B   Gynaecomastia
☐   C   Soft and small testes on palpation
☐   D   Short stature
☐   E   Low levels of follicle-stimulating hormone (FSH) and luteinising hormone (LH)

Answers on page 202

7.3   **Which of the following statements is most accurate with regard to Wilson's disease?**

☐   A   The primary defect is believed to be enhanced intestinal absorption of copper

☐   B   An alternative diagnosis should be considered if chorea occurs in the absence of Kayser–Fleischer rings

☐   C   Chronic liver disease and autoimmune haemolytic anaemia are recognised features

☐   D   Raised serum copper levels are evident at birth

☐   E   A sibling with biochemical evidence of the disease is treated only when he or she becomes symptomatic

7.4   **Which one of the following diseases has an autosomal dominant inheritance?**

☐   A   Huntington's disease
☐   B   Childhood polycystic kidney disease
☐   C   Cystic fibrosis
☐   D   Haemochromatosis
☐   E   Colour blindness

7.5   **The substitution of the amino acid valine instead of the normal glutamic acid at position 6 of the β-globin chain is the genetic abnormality encountered in which one of the following types of congenital haemolytic anaemia?**

☐   A   Sickle cell anaemia
☐   B   β-Thalassaemia
☐   C   Hereditary spherocytosis
☐   D   Glucose-6-phosphate dehydrogenase (G6PD) deficiency
☐   E   Methaemoglobinaemia

7.6   **Which one of the following inherited diseases is due to a mutation in mitochondrial DNA?**

☐   A   Alport's syndrome
☐   B   Leber's optic neuropathy
☐   C   Noonan's syndrome
☐   D   Fabry's disease
☐   E   Marfan's syndrome

7.7 **Which one of the following statements about the features of haemochromatosis is true?**

☐ A The primary defect is poor utilisation of iron by the bone marrow
☐ B Hypogonadism is caused by haemosiderin deposition in the gonads
☐ C Hepatoma is a rare complication
☐ D Clinically significant renal parenchymal disease occurs in half the patients with this condition
☐ E The diabetes mellitus is usually insulin-dependent

7.8 **Which one of the following statements about X-linked recessive disorders is true?**

☐ A A heterozygous mother will transmit the trait to half of her daughters
☐ B All the daughters born to an affected father and a normal mother will be affected
☐ C Half of the paternal uncles will be affected
☐ D All the daughters of a heterozygous mother will be carriers
☐ E All the maternal uncles will be affected

Chapter 8

HAEMATOLOGY

Questions

8.1 A retired 69-year-old man presents to the Emergency Department with a temperature of 39 °C. The white cell count (WCC) is 45 × 10⁹/l with 90% neutrophils. Which one of the following findings would be most useful for differentiating chronic myeloid leukaemia (CML) from a leukaemoid reaction?

- [ ] A Philadelphia chromosome
- [ ] B Splenic enlargement
- [ ] C Low leucocyte alkaline phosphatase score
- [ ] D Hypercellular bone marrow
- [ ] E Elevated platelet count

8.2 A 40-year-old woman presents with excessive tiredness, lethargy and breathlessness on exertion. She also complains of a sore mouth and tongue. Her serum B12 is 4 pmol/l (normal range 120–700 pmol/l). Which one of the following findings would be most suggestive of megaloblastic anaemia?

- [ ] A Hypersegmented neutrophils in the peripheral blood film
- [ ] B Atrophic gastritis
- [ ] C Pancytopenia
- [ ] D Low reticulocyte count
- [ ] E Raised lactate dehydrogenase (LDH)

8.3   A 66-year-old man presents with fatigue and excessive pallor. Investigations show his haemoglobin to be 7.7 g/dl, with a hypochromic microcytic picture; the serum ferritin is 3 µg/l (normal range 15–300 µg/l). Which one of the following statements regarding this type of anaemia is most accurate?

- ☐   A   It is commonly caused by dietary deficiency
- ☐   B   Pins and needles in the hands and feet may indicate early peripheral neuropathy
- ☐   C   Splenomegaly occurs in up to 50% of cases
- ☐   D   Koilonychia is characteristic and is rarely seen in other forms of anaemia
- ☐   E   The reticulocyte count is often elevated

8.4   Which one of the following features is most characteristic of Waldenström's macroglobulinaemia?

- ☐   A   Bone pain
- ☐   B   A monoclonal IgM peak
- ☐   C   Renal impairment
- ☐   D   Multiple osteolytic lesions
- ☐   E   Absence of immune paresis

8.5   A 23-year-old woman is referred with hypochromic microcytic anaemia. She describes heavy menstrual periods. She has a family history of β-thalassaemia trait. Which one of the following features would be most helpful for distinguishing β-thalassaemia trait from iron deficiency anaemia?

- ☐   A   Microcytosis
- ☐   B   Haemoglobin A$_2$ levels
- ☐   C   Reduced haematocrit
- ☐   D   Splenomegaly
- ☐   E   Target cells on peripheral blood examination

8.6 Which one of the following adverse effects of blood transfusion is most likely to be mediated by donor plasma proteins?

☐ A   Febrile non-haemolytic transfusion reaction (FNHTR)
☐ B   Transmission of AIDS
☐ C   Transfusion-related acute lung injury (TRALI)
☐ D   Alloimmunisation against platelets
☐ E   Transmission of cytomegalovirus (CMV)

8.7 A 30-year-old woman presents with extreme tiredness and pallor. The full blood count shows: haemoglobin 6.7 g/dl, white cell count 11.5 × 10^9/l, platelet count 535 × 10^9/l. The serum total bilirubin is significantly raised at 187 µmol/l (normal range 1–22 µmol/l); the AST and ALT are within normal limits. The reticulocyte count was five times above the normal limit. Therapeutic plasmapheresis would be considered as potentially effective if this type of anaemia was due to which one of the following conditions?

☐ A   Haemolytic anaemia associated with *Mycoplasma pneumoniae* infection
☐ B   Thalassaemia major
☐ C   Systemic lupus erythematosus- (SLE-) associated haemolytic anaemia
☐ D   Paroxysmal nocturnal haemoglobinuria (PNH)
☐ E   Aplastic anaemia

8.8 A 69-year-old woman with rheumatoid arthritis presents with bleeding from an arthrocentesis site and melaena. Blood tests show: haemoglobin 5.6 g/dl, INR 1, activated partial thromboplastin time (APTT) 94 s (normal range 30–40 s), factor VIII activity 4%, and a high factor VIII inhibitor titre of 5 Bethesda units (BU). Her medical notes show that she has had knee surgery twice before, 3 and 5 years ago, with no excessive bleeding reported. Which one of the following is the most likely cause of this patient's bleeding?

☐ A   Haemophilia A
☐ B   von Willebrand disease (vWD)
☐ C   Acquired haemophilia
☐ D   Bernard–Soulier syndrome
☐ E   Disseminated intravascular coagulation (DIC)

8.9 A 70-year-old man presents with generalised lymphadenopathy and hepatosplenomegaly. The peripheral blood film shows a WCC of 23.5 × 10⁹/l, with 70% mature lymphocytes. Which one of the following clinical findings is characteristic of this disorder?

- [ ] A   The median survival after diagnosis is 2 years
- [ ] B   T lymphocytes are the cell line in the majority of cases
- [ ] C   Bone marrow examination is essential to confirm the diagnosis
- [ ] D   Paraprotein of the IgG kappa light chain type is identified in 50% of cases
- [ ] E   It can transform to lymphoma

8.10 A pregnant 22-year-old woman presents at the Antenatal Clinic with multiple bruises around the thigh and upper arm. She is 6 months' pregnant and apart from tiredness she has no other symptoms. The full blood count (FBC) shows: haemoglobin 11.7 g/dl, white cell count 7.5 × 10⁹/l, platelet count 75 × 10⁹/l. Bone marrow examination shows abundant and large megakaryocytes. Antiplatelet antibodies are positive. Which one of the following features is characteristic of this disorder?

- [ ] A   Infants born to a woman with this condition often present with bleeding diathesis in the first 48 hours
- [ ] B   Pancytopenia is a recognised complication
- [ ] C   Leukaemic transformation occurs late in the disease
- [ ] D   Splenomegaly is found in 50% of cases
- [ ] E   Autoimmune haemolytic anaemia is a recognised association

8.11 A 62-year-old man presents with general lethargy, pallor and reduced exercise tolerance. On examination, he is found to have splenomegaly. The peripheral blood shows: haemoglobin 7.7 g/dl, white cell count $2.8 \times 10^9/l$, platelet count $45 \times 10^9/l$. A bone marrow biopsy has identified hairy cells. Which one of the following is true of this disorder?

☐ A It has a female : male preponderance of 10 : 2
☐ B Generalised lymphadenopathy is the most common presenting feature
☐ C It results in a 'dry tap' marrow aspirate despite the presence of marrow hypercellularity
☐ D It is caused by aberration in the maturation of T lymphocytes
☐ E The disease course is more aggressive than in acute leukaemias

8.12 A 14-year-old boy presents with an acute febrile illness and multiple bruises. The peripheral blood examination and bone marrow report confirm the diagnosis of acute lymphoblastic leukaemia (ALL). Which one of the following is a poor prognostic sign in this disease?

☐ A Low initial leucocyte count
☐ B Age <15 years
☐ C The presence of Philadelphia chromosome
☐ D Pre-B phenotype
☐ E cALLa type

8.13 A 44-year-old woman is admitted to hospital with overwhelming chest infection. She has had three similar admissions in the last 18 months. Howell–Jolly bodies and nucleated red blood cells are identified on peripheral blood examination. Which one of the following conditions is this patient most likely to be suffering from?

☐ A Thalassaemia
☐ B Coeliac disease
☐ C Rheumatoid arthritis
☐ D Myxoedema
☐ E Cirrhosis of the liver

8.14   A 72-year-old man presents with progressive weight loss and pallor. Examination reveals massive splenomegaly. Bone marrow examination confirms the diagnosis of myelofibrosis. Which one of the following features is most characteristic of this disorder?

☐   A   Leucoerythroblastic blood picture
☐   B   Extensive plasma cell infiltration of the bone marrow
☐   C   Multiple fragility fractures
☐   D   Rod-shaped red blood cells
☐   E   Eventual conversion to multiple myeloma

8.15   A 20-year old student is referred with an acutely painful right knee. He is known to have haemophilia A. Which one of the following statements most accurately describes this patient's condition?

☐   A   Petechiae are more common than soft-tissue bleeding
☐   B   The bleeding time is prolonged
☐   C   Factor VIII inhibitors occur in 10% of patients receiving multiple factor VIII transfusions
☐   D   Iron deficiency anaemia is a frequent and persistent problem
☐   E   Joint deformity is rare despite the fact that haemarthrosis is one of the main and recurrent manifestations

8.16   A 56-year-old woman is referred for further assessment because a recent full blood count had revealed a platelet count of 700 × 10^9/l. Which one of the following disorders may explain this blood abnormality?

☐   A   Pernicious anaemia
☐   B   Haemolytic-uraemic syndrome
☐   C   Paroxysmal nocturnal haemoglobinuria
☐   D   Iron deficiency anaemia due to blood loss
☐   E   Antiphospholipid syndrome

8.17   A 16-year-old boy who is known to have sickle cell anaemia presents with fever and headache. The FBC shows a WCC of $2.5 \times 10^9/l$ and a platelet count of $35 \times 10^9/l$. Which one of the following is the most likely cause of this patient's recent deterioration?

☐   A   Dehydration
☐   B   Respiratory syncytial virus infection
☐   C   Human parvovirus B19 infection
☐   D   Repeated blood transfusion
☐   E   *Haemophilus influenzae* septicaemia

8.18   In recent years, low molecular weight (LMW) heparins have become the standard treatment for thromboembolism. Compared with unfractionated heparin, which one of the following advantages has made them such an attractive choice?

☐   A   They do not bind antithrombin
☐   B   Their use is not associated with heparin-induced thrombocytopenia
☐   C   Their shorter half-life reduces the risk of bleeding
☐   D   They can be used safely in patients with haemorrhagic stroke
☐   E   Laboratory monitoring of activated partial thromboplastin time is not required

8.19   A 58-year-old man complains of recurrent epistaxis and recently presented with an overwhelming infection. The peripheral blood film shows: haemoglobin 6.7 g/dl, white cell count $2.5 \times 10^9/l$, platelet count $45 \times 10^9/l$. The bone marrow biopsy shows hypocellular marrow. In an attempt to find a possible underlying cause, you will consider investigating for which one of the following tumours?

☐   A   Teratoma
☐   B   Atrial myxoma
☐   C   Hypernephroma
☐   D   Thymoma
☐   E   Carcinoma of the bronchus

8.20   A 33-year-old man from Greece who is known to have
       thalassaemia is referred for assessment of possible transfusion
       haemosiderosis. He was diagnosed with thalassaemia as a child.
       He received multiple blood transfusions over the years. Which
       one of the following statements is true?

☐   A   Symptoms of iron overload usually develop once more than
        10 units of packed erythrocytes have been transfused
☐   B   Conduction defects are a frequent early symptom of cardiac
        involvement
☐   C   The diagnosis can be made by assessment of serum ferritin
        level and liver biopsy
☐   D   The treatment of choice is oral D-penicillamine (a chelating
        agent)
☐   E   Because of the associated chronic anaemia, patients with
        thalassaemia are very resistant to transfusion haemosiderosis

8.21   A 56-year-old man with chronic renal failure considered suitable
       for haemodialysis presents with retrosternal chest pain, fatigue
       and excessive pallor. The full blood count shows a haemoglobin
       concentration of 8.7 g/dl, with a normocytic and normochromic
       picture. The ECG shows T-wave inversion in leads II and III. In
       addition to anti-anginal treatment, which one of the following is
       the best way to correct his anaemia at this stage?

☐   A   Blood transfusion
☐   B   Iron infusion
☐   C   Recombinant human erythropoietin (epoeitin)
☐   D   Nandrolone decanoate
☐   E   B12 injections 3-monthly

8.22   Which one of the following bone sites is the most common site
       involved in bone metastases from carcinomata?

☐   A   Ribs
☐   B   Pelvis
☐   C   Spine
☐   D   Skull
☐   E   Long bones

8.23 **A 30-year old woman presents with excessive tiredness and lethargy. She also complains of sore mouth and tongue. The serum folate concentration is 0.5 µg/l (normal range 2.0–11.0 µg/l). Which one of the following statements is true about folic acid deficiency?**

- [ ] A Because of the high body stores of folate, it will take more than 2 years for megaloblastic anaemia to develop after complete cessation of folic acid intake
- [ ] B Methotrexate-induced folic acid deficiency can often be corrected by concomitant folic acid supplementation
- [ ] C Intestinal bacterial overgrowth is regarded as one of the common causes
- [ ] D It causes abnormal neurological findings that are indistinguishable from those associated with vitamin B12 deficiency
- [ ] E It is responsible for neural tube defects in the fetus

Chapter 9

INFECTIOUS DISEASES

Questions

9.1 A 48-year-old alcoholic presents with abdominal pain, fever and rigors. He has been passing dark-coloured urine. He is confused. Abdominal examination reveals moderate ascites, generalised tenderness and hypoactive bowel sounds. Ascitic fluid analysis reveals a total protein level of 1.1 g/dl and 3600 white cells/μl with 2448 neutrophils/μl (68%). Gram stain and culture of the ascitic fluid were negative. Which one of the following is the most likely diagnosis?

☐ A Alcoholic hepatitis
☐ B Cholangitis
☐ C Chronic pancreatitis
☐ D Septic meningitis
☐ E Spontaneous bacterial peritonitis

9.2 Which one of the following infections is caused by bacteria of the genus *Chlamydia*?

☐ A Q fever
☐ B Lyme disease
☐ C Psittacosis ornithosis
☐ D River blindness
☐ E Chagas disease

9.3   Which one of the following is characteristic of haemolytic-uraemic syndrome?

☐   A   It is more common in the elderly
☐   B   Fragmented red blood cells are seen on peripheral blood film examination
☐   C   Fever and transient cerebral disorders are frequently present
☐   D   *Escherichia coli* is isolated from the blood in more than 50% of cases
☐   E   The mortality rate has improved but remains in the region of 70%

9.4   Which one of the following statements regarding malaria is accurate?

☐   A   In *Plasmodium vivax* infection, fever and rigors usually manifest 2 days after bite from an infected mosquito
☐   B   In *P. malariae* infection, a relapse can occur even 2 years after the patient has left an area prone to malaria
☐   C   Chloroquine is generally ineffective in the treatment of *P. falciparum* infection
☐   D   Africans with sickle cell trait are more susceptible to malaria
☐   E   Blood culture is usually diagnostic

9.5   A 60-year-old woman is convalescing in hospital, 3 weeks after undergoing a total right knee replacement. She develops headache, chills and a fever of 39.2 °C. On examination, the right knee is red, hot and very tender. Synovial fluid aspirate shows growth of Gram-positive cocci. Which of the following is the most likely causative organism?

☐   A   *Staphylococcus epidermidis*
☐   B   *Pseudomonas aeruginosa*
☐   C   *Streptococcus pneumoniae*
☐   D   *Staphylococcus aureus*
☐   E   *Haemophilus influenzae*

9.6 **Which one of the following disorders is transmitted by accidental ingestion of the cyst of the parasite?**

☐ A Malaria
☐ B Hydatid disease
☐ C Trypanosomiasis
☐ D Leishmaniasis
☐ E Lyme disease

9.7 **With regard to multidrug-resistant tuberculosis (MDR-TB), which one of the following statements is accurate?**

☐ A It is usually caused by *Mycobacterium avium-intracellulare* (MAI)
☐ B MDR-TB is a phenomenon exclusive to patients with AIDS
☐ C Sputum smear for acid-fast bacilli is often negative
☐ D Resistance is most often encountered to isoniazid
☐ E Directly observed therapy has not been proved to be of any value in controlling MDR-TB

9.8 **A 74-year-old woman presents to her doctor with a painful rash that she first noticed the day before. On examination, a group of erythematous vesicles is noted over the right flank in the T10 dermatome distribution. Reasonable treatment options at this stage would include which one of the following?**

☐ A Cyclophosphamide
☐ B Aciclovir
☐ C Erythromycin
☐ D Carbamazepine
☐ E Gluten-free diet

9.9 A 21-year-old student who is taking the oral contraceptive pill develops pain and soreness around the genital area. She has just completed an elective year in the USA. On examination, there are multiple, shallow and tender ulcers on the skin and mucous membrane of the vagina. Which one of the following is the most probable diagnosis?

☐ A   Genital herpes
☐ B   Chancroid
☐ C   Granuloma inguinale
☐ D   Primary syphilis
☐ E   Lymphogranuloma venereum

9.10 A 19-year-old female university student presents with fever and headache. On examination, she is conscious but has neck stiffness. The cerebrospinal fluid Gram stain shows intracellular Gram-negative diplococci. Which of the following is the most probable diagnosis?

☐ A   Meningococcal meningitis
☐ B   *Haemophilus influenzae* meningitis
☐ C   *Streptococcus pneumoniae* meningitis
☐ D   *Listeria monocytogenes*
☐ E   *Escherichia coli* meningitis

9.11 A 70-year-old man with non-insulin-dependent diabetes mellitus (NIDDM) is admitted with pain and swelling in the left ear and face. On examination, the external ear is red, tender and swollen. There is a small amount of purulent discharge from the external auditory canal, with crust covering the skin. The left side of his face is swollen, with tenderness over the left temporal bone. Which one of the following is the most probable primary micro-organism responsible for this infection?

☐ A   *Pseudomonas aeruginosa*
☐ B   *Staphylococcus aureus*
☐ C   *Streptococcus pneumoniae*
☐ D   *Listeria monocytogenes*
☐ E   *Haemophilus influenzae*

9.12 **Which one of the following statements is true with regard to Legionnaires' disease?**

☐ A *Legionella pneumophila* is a Gram-positive rod
☐ B The urinary antigen test for *Legionella* species has low sensitivity and is not particularly specific
☐ C The infection is generally confined to immunocompromised patients
☐ D The β-lactam drugs are now regarded as the drugs of first choice against *Legionella* species
☐ E Hyponatraemia occurs significantly more often in Legionnaires' disease than in other pneumonias

9.13 **Which one of the following is true regarding indium leucocyte imaging (¹¹¹In-labelled leucocyte studies)?**

☐ A The entire body can be checked for infectious disease sites
☐ B It is used specifically to detect splenic abscess
☐ C It is very useful for differentiating between Crohn's disease and ulcerative colitis
☐ D It is often used to localise the source of active gastrointestinal bleeding
☐ E It is useful in the diagnosis of chronic lymphatic leukaemia

9.14 **Which one of the following statements about Kaposi's sarcoma (KS) is true?**

☐ A The incidence of KS in AIDS has been in progressive decline since the early 1990s
☐ B There is a 400× increased risk of KS among patients with congenital immune deficiency
☐ C Respiratory tract disease is the most common initial manifestation
☐ D In recent years the incidence of KS in AIDS in heterosexual men has exceeded that in homosexual and bisexual men
☐ E KS is rarely encountered in organ transplant patients

9.15   Which one of the following statements regarding AIDS is true?

☐   A   Oral hairy leukoplakia is caused by an underlying squamous cell carcinoma

☐   B   AIDS is the most likely diagnosis if *Mycobacterium avium-intracellulare* (MAI) is isolated from a biopsy specimen of an enlarged lymph node in an otherwise healthy individual presenting with generalised lymphadenopathy

☐   C   Sputum culture is likely to provide diagnostic results for *Pneumocystis carinii*

☐   D   Herpes simplex virus (HSV) infection is the most common cause of retinitis in AIDS

☐   E   Kaposi's sarcoma is encountered equally among homosexual and heterosexual AIDS patients

9.16   There are some important differences between the life cycles of *Plasmodium vivax* and *Plasmodium falciparum*. From the list below, which life cycle stage occurs with *P. vivax* but not with *P. falciparum* infection?

☐   A   Gametocytes
☐   B   Hypnozoites
☐   C   Schizonts
☐   D   Sporozoites
☐   E   Trophozoites

9.17   A 5-year-old boy is admitted with a temperature of 39.6 °C and a rash consisting of numerous dusky-pink macules and papules. He became unwell 6 days ago, when his mother noticed that he had a dry cough, red eyes and a temperature. The rash started 2 days prior to admission, appearing on his face initially, but then spreading to the trunk and limbs. He was in contact with a boy with a similar rash 10 days ago. There is no significant past medical history. He had not received all of his childhood immunisations because of parental concerns regarding vaccine safety. Which one of the following organisms is the likely cause of his rash?

- ☐   A   Epstein–Barr virus (EBV)
- ☐   B   Measles virus
- ☐   C   Parvovirus B19
- ☐   D   Rubella virus
- ☐   E   Mumps virus

9.18   You have been informed that an organism is growing in both the aerobic and the anaerobic blood culture bottles that you obtained from a patient yesterday. A Gram-positive coccus has been isolated, which is growing in small clusters. On further laboratory testing, it is shown to cause the coagulation of fibrinogen to a fibrin clot when added to diluted plasma in a test tube. Which of the following is the most likely organism?

- ☐   A   *Enterobacter cloacae*
- ☐   B   *Staphylococcus aureus*
- ☐   C   *Staphylococcus epidermidis*
- ☐   D   *Streptococcus pneumoniae*
- ☐   E   *Streptococcus pyogenes*

9.19   A 44-year-old woman who is taking oral prednisolone for a flare-up of her rheumatoid arthritis is planning a 6-week holiday to a remote jungle region of Latin America. She has completed her childhood vaccination programme, and had a polio booster 8 years ago. However, she has heard that she requires further travel vaccinations. Her travel agent has suggested the items listed below, but she is a bit concerned about the safety of these, given her medical history. Which one of the following vaccines do you feel poses the greatest difficulty?

☐   A   Polio
☐   B   Hepatitis A
☐   C   Tetanus
☐   D   Typhoid Vi
☐   E   Yellow fever

9.20   A 49-year-old woman is referred to you by her doctor who suspects chronic fatigue syndrome. Which one of the following features might suggest an alternative diagnosis?

☐   A   Dysphagia
☐   B   Frequent headaches
☐   C   Memory impairment
☐   D   Recurrent sore throats
☐   E   Severe myalgia

9.21   A 52-year-old man wishes to commence therapy for chronic hepatitis C virus (HCV) infection. He wishes to take a regime which has the best chance of conferring sustained virological success. Which one of the following treatment options would you recommend?

☐   A   Interferon-α alone
☐   B   Interferon-α with ribavirin
☐   C   Ribavirin alone
☐   D   Ribavirin with lamivudine
☐   E   Lamivudine alone

9.22   A 23-year-old woman received a renal transplant for chronic
         renal failure secondary to lupus nephritis 3 months ago and now
         presents with a 2-week history of fever, malaise and arthralgia.
         She takes ciclosporin and prednisolone. Examination reveals a
         temperature of 38.2 °C and cervical lymphadenopathy. The full
         blood count shows a white cell count of 3.8 × 10⁹/l, a neutrophil
         count of 1.1 × 10⁹/l, with numerous atypical lymphocytes seen on
         examination of the peripheral blood film. The renal function is
         normal but the liver enzymes are marginally elevated. Which of
         the following options is the most likely cause of this patient's
         present complaint?

☐   A   Acute transplant rejection
☐   B   Tuberculosis
☐   C   Cytomegalovirus (CMV) infection
☐   D   Infectious mononucleosis
☐   E   Kaposi's sarcoma

9.23   A 32-year-old farmer's wife presents with fever and malaise,
         feeling generally 'washed-out', and off her food. She has recently
         been helping out with lambing on the farm. On examination,
         there is generalised lymph node swelling and a palpable liver
         edge. Her white cell count is just below the normal range. What
         diagnosis fits best with this clinical picture?

☐   A   Tuberculosis
☐   B   Subacute bacterial endocarditis
☐   C   Brucellosis
☐   D   Amoebic liver abscess
☐   E   Mixed connective tissue disease

Chapter 10
NEPHROLOGY
Questions

10.1 A 19-year-old student presents with acute shortness of breath and haemoptysis. She reported left loin pain and was found to have haematuria 2 weeks ago. She is under regular review by the renal physicians for nephrotic syndrome. Ultrasound of the kidney shows left renal vein thrombosis and a computed tomography pulmonary angiogram confirms acute pulmonary embolism. Which one of the following is the most likely cause of this patient's increased tendency for developing venous thrombosis?

☐ A Factor V Leiden mutation
☐ B High levels of anticardiolipin antibodies
☐ C Protein S deficiency
☐ D Protien C deficiency
☐ E Antithrombin III deficiency

10.2 A 27-year-old car salesman is referred for further investigation of haematuria. Urinalysis reveals red blood cell casts. Further tests show proteinuria. Repeated complement levels assay shows normal values. What is the most likely histopathological diagnosis in this patient?

☐ A Post-streptococcal glomerulonephritis
☐ B Diffuse proliferative glomerulonephritis associated with systemic lupus erythematosus (SLE)
☐ C Subacute bacterial endocarditis-associated glomerulonephritis
☐ D Primary membranous glomerulonephritis
☐ E Primary type 1 mesangiocapillary glomerulonephritis

Answers on page 229

10.3   A 50-year-old man with alcoholic liver disease presents with rapid deterioration in his renal function, with a urea of 42 mmol/l and a creatinine of 700 µmol/l. Which one of the following statements best describes the hepatorenal syndrome?

- [ ]   A   It is due to glomerulonephritis-associated liver disease
- [ ]   B   Almost all patients have ascites and are usually jaundiced
- [ ]   C   Marked proteinuria is the hallmark of the disease
- [ ]   D   *Escherichia coli* is often isolated on blood culture
- [ ]   E   Complete recovery is expected in the majority of cases

10.4   A 30-year-old lorry driver is referred to the Nephrology Unit for further evaluation. He presented with acute shortness of breath. A plain chest X-ray shows pulmonary oedema. The renal profile shows a urea of 32 mmol/l and creatinine of 500 µmol/l. The presence of which one of the following features is most helpful in distinguishing chronic from acute renal failure?

- [ ]   A   Seizures
- [ ]   B   Bilateral small kidneys
- [ ]   C   Hypocalcaemia
- [ ]   D   Dilute urine with high urine sodium
- [ ]   E   Acute pulmonary oedema

10.5   A 40-year-old man is referred with multiple necrotic lesions on both his legs. He feels generally unwell and is admitted to hospital. His investigations show evidence of active glomerulonephritis. Which one of the following vasculitides has a particular association with renal involvement?

- [ ]   A   Churg–Strauss syndrome
- [ ]   B   Takayasu's arteritis
- [ ]   C   Microscopic polyangiitis
- [ ]   D   Cryoglobulinaemic vasculitis
- [ ]   E   Henoch–Schönlein purpura

10.6   A 30-year-old man is referred because of recent-onset haemoptysis and impaired renal function. The histopathology and immunofluorescent studies confirm the diagnosis of Goodpasture's syndrome. Which one of the following is the most characteristic feature of this disorder?

☐   A   Autosomal recessive inheritance
☐   B   Young males are particularly affected
☐   C   Linear deposits at the glomerular basement membrane on indirect immunofluorescent testing
☐   D   Pulmonary haemorrhage usually precedes renal involvement
☐   E   Vasculitic skin rash early in the disease

10.7   Which one of the following statements about retroperitoneal fibrosis is true?

☐   A   Low back pain is the most common presenting symptom
☐   B   Bilateral swelling of the legs is often due to inferior vena caval obstruction
☐   C   Pizotifen (migraine treatment) is implicated in causing a similar condition
☐   D   Renal failure is due to fibrous tissue infiltrating the kidneys
☐   E   Hashimoto's thyroiditis is a recognised association

10.8   Which one of the following features is characteristic of Bartter's syndrome?

☐   A   Hypokalaemia with hypertension
☐   B   Reduced urinary excretion of potassium and chloride
☐   C   Good response to angiotensin-converting enzyme inhibitors
☐   D   Low renin and aldosterone
☐   E   Hyperplasia of the juxtaglomerular apparatus

10.9   A 47-year-old man is referred for further assessment because of a finding of abnormal renal function on three separate occasions in the last year. The last test shows a urea of 22 mmol/l and creatinine of 250 μmol/l. Ultrasound studies demonstrate large kidneys. Which one of the following conditions is the most likely diagnosis?

☐   A   Amyloidosis
☐   B   Hypertensive nephrosclerosis
☐   C   Membranous glomerulonephritis
☐   D   Systemic sclerosis
☐   E   Analgesic nephropathy

10.10 A 10-year-old boy is hospitalised because of recent melaena and fever (38 °C). He also has arthralgia involving the knees and ankles. On examination, he has a purpuric rash on his legs. Urinalysis reveals proteinuria with microscopic haematuria. A biopsy of the purpuric lesion reveals leucocytoclastic vasculitis in the small vessels. Which one of the following statements about this boy's illness is true?

☐   A   The purpuric skin rash is due to associated thrombocytopenia
☐   B   Active urinary sediment with red blood cell casts indicates glomerulonephritis
☐   C   Identification of anti-glomerular basement membrane antibodies would be expected in 50% of cases
☐   D   Perinuclear-staining anti-neutrophil cytoplasmic antibody (pANCA) is positive in two-thirds of cases
☐   E   Renal granulomas are pathognomonic

10.11 A 40-year-old woman is referred with polyuria. She wakes up more than three times at night to pass water; her 24-hour urine volume is found to be 5 litres. Blood tests, including glucose and renal function tests, are normal. Diabetes insipidus is the primary diagnostic possibility but because of a past medical history of schizophrenia, psychogenic polydypsia is also being considered. Which one of the following tests would be most helpful for differentiating between these disorders?

- [ ] A   Plasma osmolality
- [ ] B   Renal ultrasound
- [ ] C   Psychiatric assessment
- [ ] D   Urine specific gravity
- [ ] E   Magnetic resonance imaging (MRI) of the pituitary gland

10.12 A 33-year-old man is referred with acute shortness of breath and oliguria. His urea is 34 mmol/l and the creatinine is 570 μmol/l. Urinalysis using polarised microscopy reveals large numbers of needle-shaped crystals. Which one of the following drugs is most likely to be the cause of this patient's sudden deterioration?

- [ ] A   Allopurinol
- [ ] B   Penicillin antibiotics
- [ ] C   Aciclovir
- [ ] D   Angiotensin-converting enzyme (ACE) inhibitors
- [ ] E   Gentamicin

10.13 Which one of the following statements about general urine examination is true?

- [ ] A   Hyaline casts indicate end-stage renal failure
- [ ] B   Green urine colour may be due to urinary tract infection caused by *Escherichia coli*
- [ ] C   Granular casts are often associated with renal parenchymal disease
- [ ] D   Dysmorphic red blood cells indicate bladder disease
- [ ] E   Fat globules are seen in pyelonephritis

Answers on pages 232–234

10.14 A 45-year-old man is admitted with acute renal failure of undetermined aetiology. His creatinine is 1564 µmol/l and his urea is 76 mmol/l. His blood pressure is 200/110 mmHg; he is oliguric; and he has pulmonary oedema confirmed on chest X-ray. A dual-lumen dialysis line is inserted into his right subclavian vein, and the position is confirmed by chest X-ray. He is urgently commenced on haemodialysis, in a recumbent position, with a target weight loss of 1.5 kg. One hour into dialysis, he begins to complain of nausea, headache and blurred vision. Shortly afterwards, he becomes confused and disorientated; his blood pressure is 180/100 mmHg. Which one of the following is the most likely explanation?

- ☐ A   Air embolism
- ☐ B   Reaction to hypotonic dialysate
- ☐ C   Dysequilibrium syndrome
- ☐ D   Pericardial tamponade
- ☐ E   Intravascular volume contraction resulting from rapid ultrafiltration

10.15 Wilms' tumour is most strongly associated with which one of the following aetiological factors?

- ☐ A   Cadmium exposure
- ☐ B   Smoking
- ☐ C   Naphthylamine
- ☐ D   A deletion on the short arm of chromosome 11
- ☐ E   Balkan nephropathy

10.16 A 32-year-old man is diagnosed with hypertension. Which one of the following features would suggest that he has an underlying renal artery stenosis?

- ☐ A   Proximal muscle weakness
- ☐ B   Wheezing, flushing and diarrhoea
- ☐ C   Truncal obesity and easy bruising
- ☐ D   Plethoric face and splenomegaly
- ☐ E   Multiple *café au lait* spots and subcutaneous nodules

10.17 A 50-year-old woman is being investigated for a cavity lesion in the lung and glomerulonephritis. A biopsy from the kidney confirms the diagnosis of Wegener's granulomatosis. Which one of the following would be a poor prognostic factor in this patient?

- A Female sex
- B Anti-neutrophil cytoplasmic antibody (cANCA) positivity
- C Pulmonary disease
- D Vasculitic skin rash
- E Renal involvement

10.18 A pregnant 23-year-old woman who is complaining of general fatigue is referred for further investigation. Which one of the following abnormal test results is most likely to be associated with an underlying pathological disorder?

- A Glycosuria
- B Haematuria
- C Ketonuria
- D Plasma osmolality of 277 mosmol/kg
- E Ureteral dilatation

10.19 A patient on peritoneal dialysis presents with a 1-week history of abdominal pain. She has been on dialysis for 2 years and also has a history of coronary artery disease. Clinically, her abdomen is rigid and distended, with absent bowel sounds; blood pressure 85/50 mmHg; pulse rate 120 bpm. The dialysate appears very cloudy. Culture of the dialysis fluid reveals a mixed growth of *Escherichia coli, Bacteroides* spp. and *Enterobacter* spp. What is the most likely cause of this presentation?

- A Acute pancreatitis
- B Diverticulitis
- C Myocardial infarction
- D Primary peritoneal-dialysis peritonitis
- E Ulcerative colitis

10.20 You are asked by your orthopaedic colleagues to review a
28-year-old victim of blunt trauma after a motorcycle accident.
He has suffered extensive lower limb damage and requires large
amounts of analgesia. The orthopaedic surgeons are concerned
about his blood results: his potassium some hours after the
accident is 6.7 mmol/l; the calcium is 2.05 mmol/l. His urine is
positive for blood on dipstick urinalysis. What diagnosis fits best
with this clinical picture?

☐   A   Acute sepsis
☐   B   Hypovolaemia leading to prerenal failure
☐   C   Rhabdomyolysis
☐   D   Direct renal trauma with perinephric haematoma
☐   E   Analgesic nephropathy

Answers on page 237

Chapter 11
NEUROLOGY
Questions

11.1 A 30-year-old woman presents to the Emergency Department at 9 pm with severe headache. Two hours earlier she had felt as if she was hit on the back of the head and she then experienced severe occipital headache and vomiting. A diagnosis of subarachnoid haemorrhage is suspected. Urgent computed tomography (CT) scan of the brain is normal. Which one of the following is the most appropriate next step in the management?

☐ A Reassure and discharge after prescribing strong painkillers
☐ B Observe in hospital and repeat the CT brain scan the next morning
☐ C Perform a lumbar puncture and cerebrospinal fluid (CSF) analysis immediately
☐ D Observe in hospital and delay lumbar puncture and CSF analysis until the next morning
☐ E Arrange urgent magnetic resonance imaging (MRI) of the brain

11.2 A 70-year-old woman is referred for urgent assessment of double vision. She describes having to cover one eye with her hand to focus. Which one of the following findings would be most suggestive of myasthenia gravis?

☐ A Symmetrical external ocular muscle weakness
☐ B Preserved pupillary light reflex with absent accommodation reflex
☐ C Thymoma on computed tomography scan of the chest
☐ D Elevated creatine kinase
☐ E Proptosis

11.3 A 30-year-old care assistant presents with a high temperature and severe pain and swelling in the left side of his face. He claims that this happened 2 days after he tried to squeeze a small boil in his left nostril. Which one of the following features would be most typical of cavernous sinus thrombosis?

- A   Double vision on looking upwards
- B   Papilloedema as an early feature
- C   Ipsilateral lower motor facial nerve palsy
- D   Loss of pinprick sensation around the chin area
- E   Difficulty in swallowing

11.4 A 61-year-old man presents to the Emergency Department with frequent falls and a fluctuating level of consciousness. His wife claims that it all started when he slipped and banged his head while washing his car 3 days earlier. Which one of the following statements is most accurate about chronic subdural haematoma?

- A   The trauma to the head is usually minor and often forgotten by the patient
- B   Neck stiffness is an early feature
- C   Headache is often absent
- D   Lumbar puncture and cerebrospinal fluid analysis should be done immediately on patient arrival
- E   Injury to the middle meningeal artery is the usual cause of the haematoma

11.5 Which one of the following structures within the central nervous system is pain-sensitive?

- A   Pia mater
- B   Dura mater
- C   IInd cranial nerve
- D   Parietal lobe brain tissue
- E   Occipital lobe brain tissue

11.6 A 45-year-old classroom assistant is complaining of weakness and paraesthesiae in both upper and lower limbs. She has noticed an electric shock-like sensation when she bends her neck suddenly downwards. She has had to give up her job. Her serum B12 levels are reduced. Which one of the following neurological findings is most helpful in differentiating subacute combined degeneration of the cord from multiple sclerosis?

☐ A Bilateral Babinski sign
☐ B Absent ankle jerk
☐ C Optic atrophy
☐ D 'Barber's chair' sign
☐ E Ataxia

11.7 A 69-year-old man is referred with tremor in both hands. He has started to drop things and is not able to drink from a cup. His doctor thinks that he might have either Parkinson's disease or essential tremor. Which one of the following features is more suggestive of essential tremor?

☐ A It is often associated with cogwheel rigidity
☐ B It improves with intentional movement
☐ C It is made worse by alcohol
☐ D It has a strong familial tendency
☐ E It has a tendency to improve with age

11.8 A 50-year-old woman with diabetes mellitus presents with backache and inability to walk unaided. This came on suddenly, while she was trying to lift her shopping bag from the car boot. Which one of the following is most suggestive of a lesion of the sciatic nerve?

☐ A Absent knee tendon jerk
☐ B Foot drop
☐ C Inability to flex the hip
☐ D Decreased sensation on the anterior thigh and medial leg
☐ E Intervertebral disc prolapse at L2/L3 level

11.9 A postmortem brain examination is being carried out on a 72-year-old man who had Parkinson's disease. He died from overwhelming chest infection. Which one of the following pathological brain-tissue abnormalities would you expect to find in this patient?

- ☐ A Mallory bodies
- ☐ B Lewy bodies
- ☐ C Neurofibrillary tangles
- ☐ D Pick bodies
- ☐ E Negri bodies

11.10 Chorea is a recognised feature of which one of the following?

- ☐ A Wilson's disease
- ☐ B Multiple myeloma
- ☐ C Nebulised salbutamol
- ☐ D Motor neurone disease
- ☐ E Haemochromatosis

11.11 Autonomic neuropathy is a recognised feature in which one of the following conditions?

- ☐ A Shy–Drager syndrome
- ☐ B Dermatomyositis
- ☐ C B12 deficiency
- ☐ D Multiple sclerosis
- ☐ E Myasthenia gravis

11.12 A 32-year-old woman is referred with a 2-week history of blurred vision, unsteady gait and numbness in the right hand. She has experienced several similar short-lived attacks in the past. The brain magnetic resonance imaging scan shows multiple lesions in the white matter in the periventricular area and the cerebellum, with no surrounding oedema. Which one of the following is the most probable diagnosis?

- [ ] A Thrombophilia with multiple cerebral infarcts
- [ ] B Syringomyelia
- [ ] C Metastatic tumour
- [ ] D Multiple sclerosis
- [ ] E Amyotrophic lateral sclerosis

11.13 A 40-year-old woman with paraplegia is referred for further evaluation. The magnetic resonance imaging scan of the cervical spine shows a fluid-filled syrinx and widening of the spinal cord. Which one of the following statements about syringomyelia/syringobulbia is true?

- [ ] A It is almost always associated with craniocervical malformations
- [ ] B There is loss of pain and position sense, with preservation of touch and temperature sensations
- [ ] C There is a bilateral Babinski sign
- [ ] D The syrinx is often confined to the thoracolumbar part of the spinal cord
- [ ] E There is hypertonia and exaggerated reflexes in the upper arms

11.14 A 40-year-old man has come to the Emergency Department complaining of intense headache of 2 hours' duration. The pain is localised around the right eye and is associated with tearing and redness of the eye. The patient says that he has had several similar episodes over the last year and that these episodes occurred every day for a few weeks at a time, at a rate of one to three attacks a day, each lasting for 1–2 hours, and frequently at night. Often, the attacks stop after 4–6 weeks. He lost his job in a bank 6 months ago and has noticed an increase in the intensity of the pain since. Examination reveals drooping of the eyelid and a small pupil on the right side. Which one of the following is the most probable diagnosis?

- [ ] A   Migraine
- [ ] B   Tension-type headache
- [ ] C   Iritis-associated headache
- [ ] D   Cerebral tumour
- [ ] E   Cluster headache

11.15 A 70-year-old-man arrives at the Emergency Department an hour after he felt light-headed and collapsed to the ground. He told the two paramedics who accompanied him that he has double vision whenever he looks to the right. On examination, he is conscious and alert, and there is diplopia, ptosis and a dilated pupil on the left. He also has a right hemiplegia. Occlusion of which one of the following arteries is responsible for the neurological deficits in this patient?

- [ ] A   A branch of the basilar artery
- [ ] B   Posterior cerebral artery
- [ ] C   Anterior cerebral artery
- [ ] D   Middle cerebral artery
- [ ] E   Vertebral artery

11.16 A 33-year-old-female teacher presents with sudden onset of weakness, numbness and paraesthesiae in the right leg. She has an electric shock-like feeling from the neck down the spine whenever she bends her head forwards. She had a similar attack 6 months ago affecting the left leg, which resolved spontaneously 2 weeks later. She denies any history of fits but her 26-year-old brother has epilepsy. On examination, there is evidence of profound weakness and reduced pinprick sensation in the right leg, and upgoing toes bilaterally. There is also horizontal nystagmus on looking to the right. Which one of the following would be the most appropriate test at this stage?

- A Nerve conduction studies (NCS)
- B Visual-evoked potentials (VEPs)
- C Electromyography (EMG)
- D Polysomnography
- E Electroencephalography (EEG)

11.17 A 60-year-old man is referred for urgent assessment. He is very concerned because he has fallen twice at the sink while splashing water over his face. He also claims that he loses his balance whenever he tries to pull his shirt over his head. Examination reveals a stamping gait. The presence of which one of the following clinical signs would be most helpful in establishing the diagnosis?

- A Small irregular pupil
- B Weakness and muscle fasciculation
- C Pill-rolling tremor
- D Nystagmus
- E Grasp reflex

11.18 Which one of the following disorders is a human prion disease?

- A Parkinson's disease
- B Creutzfeldt–Jakob disease
- C Huntington's disease
- D Alzheimer's disease
- E Progressive multifocal leucoencephalopathy

11.19 Elevated cerebrospinal fluid gamma-globulin concentration has been described in which one of the following conditions?

- [ ] A Myasthenia gravis
- [ ] B Lewy body dementia
- [ ] C Motor neurone disease
- [ ] D Multiple sclerosis
- [ ] E Cerebrovascular accident

11.20 You have been asked to give advice to a 46-year-old woman who has just had a computed tomography scan of the brain for the investigation of long-standing headache. The brain scan shows an empty sella. Which one of the following statements about this condition is true?

- [ ] A The pituitary gland is congenitally absent
- [ ] B Cerebrospinal fluid rhinorrhoea is a recognised presenting feature
- [ ] C It is more common in patients with anorexia nervosa
- [ ] D Raised intracranial pressure is a constant feature
- [ ] E Normal pituitary hormone evaluation excludes the disorder

11.21 An obese 30-year-old teacher, who is otherwise healthy, is being investigated for long-standing persistent headache. She has bilateral papilloedema. The computed tomography brain scan was generally normal, but a small (slit-like) lateral ventricle was noted. The cerebrospinal fluid pressure is raised. Which one of the following conditions is she most likely to be suffering from?

- [ ] A Benign intracranial hypertension
- [ ] B Aqueduct canal obstruction
- [ ] C Subdural haematoma
- [ ] D Normal-pressure hydrocephalus
- [ ] E Subarachnoid haemorrhage

11.22 A 19-year-old car mechanic has been admitted with weakness in both upper and lower limbs. He was well until last week. The finding of which one of the following features would be suggestive of Guillain–Barré syndrome?

- ☐ A Distal more than proximal muscle weakness
- ☐ B Hyper-reflexia
- ☐ C Raised cerebrospinal fluid cell count
- ☐ D Urinary incontinence
- ☐ E Segmental demyelination on nerve conduction studies

11.23 A 35-year-old national rugby player presents with rapidly progressive weakness in the right arm. He explains that he experienced severe left-sided headache yesterday, soon after he finished a training session. Examination reveals a right upper motor neurone facial weakness and a poor hand-grip on the right. On closer assessment, drooping of the left eyelid and a small left pupil are evident. The retina, optic disc and eye movements are normal in both eyes. Which one of the following is the most likely diagnosis?

- ☐ A Temporal arteritis
- ☐ B Myasthenia gravis
- ☐ C Carotid artery dissection
- ☐ D Posterior communicating artery aneurysm
- ☐ E Pancoast tumour

11.24 A 34-year-old professional dancer is referred for a neurological opinion. She first noticed difficulty in performing due to loss of balance and weakness in her right leg, and had to stop dancing 3 months ago. She now walks with a stick. You suspect multiple sclerosis as a possible diagnosis: which one of the following statements about this disease is true?

- ☐ A Symptoms are worse in cold weather
- ☐ B Pregnancy has no ill effects on the course of the disease
- ☐ C Bilateral facial nerve palsy occurs in 50% of cases
- ☐ D A predominance of sensory symptoms at presentation carries a far worse prognosis
- ☐ E Interferon-α has no role in the treatment

Answers on pages 246–248

11.25 A 48-year-old diabetic man is admitted after he suddenly collapsed at home. He had been speaking normally to his wife just beforehand. He is unconscious, with a Glasgow Coma Scale (GCS) score of 3. He has bilateral extensor plantar responses. The gaze is dysconjugate and his right eye is deviated laterally. The right pupil is larger than the left and is unresponsive to light. Which one of the following is the most likely cause of his coma?

- [ ] A   Temporal lobe haematoma with brain swelling
- [ ] B   Pontine infarction
- [ ] C   Pontine haemorrhage
- [ ] D   Hypoglycaemic coma
- [ ] E   Diabetic ketoacidosis

Answers on page 249

Chapter 12

OPHTHALMOLOGY

Questions

12.1 **The presence of which one of the following features is most helpful in differentiating optic neuritis from papilloedema?**

☐ A Haemorrhage around the optic disc area
☐ B Swelling of the optic disc on ophthalmoscopic examination of the retina
☐ C Central scotoma on perimetry
☐ D Diplopia
☐ E Hemianopia

12.2 **Altitudinal hemianopia would be a cardinal feature in which one of the following patients?**

☐ A A man who denies that he is blind
☐ B A 72-year-old woman with macular degeneration
☐ C A 70-year-old woman with headache, vomiting and swelling of the optic disc
☐ D A 74-year-old man with multiple cholesterol emboli on fundoscopy
☐ E A man with coarse facial features, large lips and spade-like hands

Answers on page 250

12.3 A 60-year-old man presents with a 1-week history of painless diplopia, which he first noticed when reading. The images are constantly horizontally and vertically separated, although he comments that the degree of separation varies. On examination, the visual acuity is 6/6 in both eyes. There is no pupil abnormality. There is a left ptosis, partially covering the pupil, and reduced abduction and depression of the left eye, both in abduction and adduction, with other ocular movements being normal. There is no other abnormality on general examination. Which one of the following is the most likely diagnosis?

- [ ] A   Sympathetic plexus lesion
- [ ] B   VIth cranial nerve palsy
- [ ] C   IIIrd cranial nerve palsy
- [ ] D   IVth cranial nerve palsy
- [ ] E   Ocular myasthenia gravis

12.4 A 22-year-old man with ulcerative colitis and chronic lower back pain has a red painful eye. Which one of the following features is likely to be present on examination of the eyes?

- [ ] A   Purulent discharge
- [ ] B   Photophobia on ophthalmoscopy
- [ ] C   A dilated pupil
- [ ] D   Profound visual loss
- [ ] E   Retinal haemorrhages

12.5 A 62-year-old man presents with episodic total loss of vision in one eye. What is the most appropriate investigation?

- [ ] A   Chest X-ray
- [ ] B   Fluorescein angiography
- [ ] C   Electrocardiography
- [ ] D   Magnetic resonance imaging brain scan
- [ ] E   Carotid Doppler

12.6 A 46-year-old diabetic man attending the Diabetic Clinic for a regular review is found to have reduced visual acuity. During a telephone referral to the Eye Clinic, the ophthalmologist asks if the patient has any risk factors for macular oedema. Which one of the following features should the referring physician bring to her attention?

☐ A Background diabetic retinopathy
☐ B Low glycosylated haemoglobin
☐ C Hypercholesterolaemia
☐ D Proteinuria
☐ E Peripheral vascular disease

12.7 A 26-year-old man presents with sudden onset of headache and double vision. The Emergency Department doctor diagnoses a IIIrd (oculomotor) nerve palsy. Which of the following is the most likely cause?

☐ A Posterior communicating artery aneurysm
☐ B Acoustic neuroma
☐ C Diabetes mellitus
☐ D Extradural haematoma
☐ E Ophthalmoplegic migraine

12.8 A 20-year-old woman presents with gradually reducing vision in her left eye of 2 weeks' duration. The visual acuities are 6/4 (right eye) and 6/36 (left eye). The left pupil reacts sluggishly and the consensual pupillary reaction in the right eye is also sluggish. The optic discs are normal. She describes having a similar episode 18 months ago, which resolved spontaneously 3 weeks later. What is the most likely diagnosis?

☐ A Cerebral tumour
☐ B Holmes–Adie pupil
☐ C Factitious visual loss
☐ D Parinaud's syndrome
☐ E Retrobulbar neuritis

12.9   A 45-year-old man who has been having syncopal episodes has been found to have heart block. He is referred to the Eye Clinic because the medical senior house officer noticed that he has limited eye movements. Which one of the following retinal findings may be related to the cardiac problem?

- ☐   A   Myopic degeneration
- ☐   B   Papilloedema
- ☐   C   Old choroidoretinitis
- ☐   D   Retinitis pigmentosa
- ☐   E   Macular degeneration

12.10   A 70-year-old woman presents with sudden loss of vision in one eye. Which of the following investigation findings most strongly supports a diagnosis of temporal arteritis?

- ☐   A   An erythrocyte sedimentation rate of 40 mm/hour
- ☐   B   An abnormal C-reactive protein level
- ☐   C   Giant-cell infiltrate in a temporal artery biopsy
- ☐   D   Homonymous hemianopia on visual field testing
- ☐   E   Positive TPHA

Answers on page 253

Chapter 13

PSYCHIATRY

Questions

13.1 A 62-year-old woman presents with a 6-month history of persistent hiccups. She is very distressed and claims that various types of treatment have failed to control the problem. You suspect that she may be suffering from psychogenic hiccups. Which one of the following features would be most likely to confirm your suspicion?

- [ ] A   Failure to respond to standard treatment
- [ ] B   The hiccups stop when she is asleep
- [ ] C   The patient exhibits features of distress and frustration
- [ ] D   Female gender
- [ ] E   Failure to respond to a Valsalva manoeuvre

13.2 Which one of the following features is most helpful in distinguishing dementia from severe depression?

- [ ] A   Persistent headache
- [ ] B   Weight loss
- [ ] C   Poor attention span
- [ ] D   Grasp reflex
- [ ] E   Social withdrawal

Answers on page 254

13.3   The risk of suicide is highest in which one of the following individuals?

☐   A   A 45-year-old woman with a history of suicide attempts
☐   B   A married man with two children
☐   C   A 50-year-old man with a history of suicide attempts
☐   D   A 30-year-old man recently diagnosed HIV-positive
☐   E   A 25-year-old woman with a history of drug overdoses

13.4   Which one of the following statements about obsessive–compulsive disorder (OCD) is accurate?

☐   A   A feeling of guilt is the core abnormal behaviour that drives the compulsions
☐   B   Thought insertion and compulsive acts are the essential features
☐   C   The patient derives pleasure from the experience
☐   D   The disorder may follow group A β-haemolytic streptococcal pharyngitis
☐   E   Major tranquillisers are the mainstay of treatment

13.5   A 28-year-old woman is admitted for investigation of recurrent epileptic fits. She is a known epileptic and has been taking phenytoin for 5 years, but her fits are not controlled. During her stay in hospital, the on-call doctor discovers that he is able to make the patient respond to verbal commands during a fit and he thinks that the fits he has witnessed have probably been psychogenic non-epileptic seizures (pseudoseizures). The presence of which one of the following features would be most helpful in establishing a diagnosis of genuine epileptic fits?

☐   A   Urinary incontinence
☐   B   Tongue biting
☐   C   Pelvic thrusting
☐   D   A history of two previous admissions with status epilepticus
☐   E   A family history of epilepsy (sister)

13.6 An 18-year-old man seen in the Out-patients Department with his mother complains that he is 'slow off the mark', has problems interacting with others and has difficulty concentrating. When you examine him you discover a high-arched palate, mitral valve prolapse, joint laxity, strabismus and large ears. Which one of the following investigations would be most useful in reaching a diagnosis?

- ☐ A Chromosomal analysis
- ☐ B Karyotyping
- ☐ C Computed tomography scan of his head
- ☐ D Urinary homocystine
- ☐ E Urinary excretion of hydroxyproline

13.7 Which one of the following fits best with a diagnosis of tardive dyskinesia?

- ☐ A Fixed contortions of the muscles of the head, neck and upper limbs
- ☐ B Symptoms occurring within a few days of administration of an antipsychotic drug
- ☐ C Abnormal involuntary movements, typically choreoathetoid, which are usually complex, rapid and stereotyped
- ☐ D Muscular rigidity, tremor and bradykinesia
- ☐ E It is always reversible

13.8 A 50-year-old man presents following the death of his wife. Which one of the following is going to heighten your suspicion of an abnormal grief reaction?

- ☐ A A brief episode of seeing the dead person
- ☐ B Poor concentration
- ☐ C Poor memory
- ☐ D Delayed or absent grief
- ☐ E Searching for the deceased

Answers on pages 255–258

13.9   A 45-year-old man with a history of paranoid schizophrenia was brought to the Emergency Department by the police as he has been 'behaving bizarrely'. There were no psychiatric beds available. He was admitted to the Medical Short-Stay Unit and received continuous monitoring from a psychiatric nurse. After a night's sleep he appeared settled and co-operative but during the day he has become extremely agitated. He screams that he can see 'people crawling all over the walls'. He looks terrified and highly distractable and gazes intermittently at the walls. At times he appears drowsy and at other times he is hyper-alert. He is disorientated in time and place, but not person. A full physical examination is impossible but he looks tremulous, is sweating profusely and staggers across the cubicle with an ataxic gait. Which one of the following is the most likely diagnosis?

- [ ] A   Exacerbation of his psychotic illness
- [ ] B   Delirium due to drug or alcohol withdrawal
- [ ] C   Drug-induced psychosis
- [ ] D   Head injury
- [ ] E   Neuroleptic malignant syndrome

13.10 A 34-year-old man presents to the Emergency Department complaining that he has had an electrical chip inserted in his head which is giving him 'great power' and sending him messages that he is 'The One'. He also claims that his legs are 'moved by the great force'. These experiences began about 9 months ago but only became troubling in the past few days. He appears slightly perplexed and concerned. However, he is settled and sits quietly in the cubicle while awaiting further assessment. Which one of the following is the most likely underlying diagnosis?

- [ ] A   Bipolar affective disorder
- [ ] B   Paranoid schizophrenia
- [ ] C   Drug-induced psychosis
- [ ] D   Cotard's syndrome
- [ ] E   Organic psychotic disorder

13.11 A 70-year-old man is brought to the Psychiatric Out-patients Clinic by his son. The son complains that his father's personality has changed completely over the past year. Even at best, he is forgetful and 'switched off'; at worst, he is drowsy and unresponsive. He is particularly concerned that his father has claimed to 'see things that aren't really there'. Over the past few weeks his father has also been tripping a lot on the carpet and is no longer safe on the stairs when going up to his bedroom unaccompanied. The family doctor gave the patient a small dose of a neuroleptic which 'made things a million times worse'. On examination, he has an inexpressive face, with a mild resting tremor and some axial rigidity. There are no other focal neurological signs. On mini mental state examination, he scores 20/30. Which one of the following is the most likely primary brain pathology?

- A   Neurofibrillary tangles
- B   Normal brain
- C   Multiple infarcts in the grey matter
- D   Lewy bodies
- E   Pick bodies

13.12 A 25-year-old man is started on chlorpromazine after being diagnosed as suffering from paranoid schizophrenia. Two months later he is seen in the clinic as an emergency because his friends are concerned that there has been an apparent deterioration in his mental state. The patient complains of an extremely distressing sense of restlessness and a complete inability to remain still. On examination, he shifts constantly in his chair and fidgets with his coat. There is a slight increase in tone on his right side and a detectable resting tremor in his hands. He describes some vague feelings of 'being watched' but there are no other psychotic symptoms elicited. Which one of the following is the most likely diagnosis?

- A   Acute dystonic reaction due to chlorpromazine
- B   Breakthrough of his psychotic symptoms
- C   Akathisia
- D   Tardive dyskinesia
- E   Tardive dystonia

Chapter 14

RESPIRATORY MEDICINE

Questions

14.1 A 50-year-old man presents with increasing shortness of breath. He is centrally cyanosed and wheezes are audible. Which one of the following statements about this patient's condition is accurate?

- [ ] A The PaO_2 at its best is not above 50 mmHg (7 kPa)
- [ ] B In methaemoglobinaemia, the PaO_2 is never above 50 mmHg (7 kPa)
- [ ] C The expected reduced haemoglobin level is around 3 g/dl
- [ ] D The blue tinge of the skin and mucous membranes is due to carbon dioxide (CO_2) retention
- [ ] E Oxygen (O_2) therapy, should be avoided as it may worsen hypercapnia

14.2 A 30-year-old housewife presents at the Emergency Department with left pleuritic chest pain and haemoptysis. She arrived in the country after a long-haul flight earlier in the day. Which one of the following clinical findings is most suggestive of pulmonary embolism?

- [ ] A Spiking temperature of 39 °C lasting more than 1 week
- [ ] B Haemoptysis of more than 5 ml with a negative chest X-ray
- [ ] C Chest pain worse on deep breathing and a respiratory rate of 26 breaths/minute
- [ ] D Recurrent previous chest pain in the same location
- [ ] E Chest pain on lying flat

Answers on page 262

14.3   **A 36-year-old bookkeeper is referred for further assessment because of increasing shortness of breath. The pulmonary function tests show a low FEV$_1$ and normal TLCO. Which one of the following conditions is most likely to be responsible for this patient's shortness of breath?**

☐   A   Asthma
☐   B   Emphysema
☐   C   Sarcoidosis
☐   D   Pulmonary embolism
☐   E   Fibrosing alveolitis

14.4   **A 24-year-old woman who is 12 weeks' pregnant presents to the Emergency Department with pain and swelling in the left leg. The left leg veins ultrasound study confirms deep venous thrombosis (DVT). Which one of the following statements is true?**

☐   A   The majority of DVTs in pregnancy are found in the right leg
☐   B   The vast majority of DVTs in pregnancy are found in calf veins
☐   C   More than 50% of cases are treated on the basis of clinical suspicion, without the need for objective tests
☐   D   Six weeks of postpartum warfarin therapy is recommended after completion of anticoagulation during the pregnancy
☐   E   Low molecular weight (LMW) heparins carry the risk of teratogenic effects and should be avoided if pregnancy is suspected

14.5   **A 27-year-old drug addict is admitted to the Intensive Care Unit with respiratory failure. Bronchoalveolar lavage analysis demonstrates heavy colonisation with *Pneumocystis carinii*. Which one of the following is most accurate with regard to this condition?**

☐   A   It occurs exclusively in AIDS
☐   B   Pleural effusion is frequently bilateral
☐   C   Auscultation of the lungs usually reveals no abnormality
☐   D   Blood culture is positive in a third of cases
☐   E   Metronidazole is the treatment of choice

14.6 A 28-year-old man is admitted with chest infection. He is known
to have cystic fibrosis. He is given antibiotics and undergoes
postural drainage in the Physiotherapy Department. Which one
of the following features is most characteristic of this condition?

☐ A Autosomal dominant inheritance
☐ B Pancreatic insufficiency is almost always identified in adult
patients
☐ C *Pseudomonas cepacia* is the most frequent organism isolated
from sputum
☐ D Family members who carry the gene are at risk of developing
mild recurrent bronchitis
☐ E Patients will typically have reduced levels of sodium and
chloride in the sweat

14.7 A 28-year-old Afro-Caribbean nurse has developed painful
nodules on the shins of both legs. She has a low-grade fever and
has lost 5 kg in weight in the 2 months prior to her presentation.
Her chest X-ray shows bilateral hilar lymphadenopathy. What is
the most likely outcome of this patient's illness?

☐ A Complete remission after an appropriate course of steroid and
cytotoxic drugs
☐ B Complete remission without any specific treatment
☐ C Complete remission initially, but soon interrupted by
increasingly frequent relapses
☐ D Development of diffuse reticulonodular changes in the lung
and progressive shortness of breath
☐ E Generalised lymphadenopathy and progressive wasting over
5–10 years

14.8   A 68-year-old woman complains of weight loss, a gradual decline in exercise tolerance and shortness of breath. Chest X-rays show an enlarged right hilum. Bronchoscopy and biopsy confirm the diagnosis of small-cell bronchial carcinoma. Which one of the following is most characteristic of this condition?

☐   A   There is usually a history of prior asbestos exposure
☐   B   It may be associated with hyponatraemia
☐   C   The cancer cell origin is from small lymphocytes (hence 'small-cell')
☐   D   It has a better prognosis than other bronchial cancers
☐   E   Surgery is often the only definitive treatment

14.9   Which one of the following statements about exercise-induced asthma is accurate?

☐   A   It is more common in adults than in children
☐   B   It is worse in summer than in winter
☐   C   Patients are more reactive to grass pollens than other asthmatics
☐   D   Exacerbations are related to cooling of the airway
☐   E   Inhaled steroids bring acute attacks under control within 60–90 minutes

14.10   A 30-year-old farmer is referred with a persistent dry cough and dyspnoea. The chest X-ray reveals multiple pulmonary infiltrates and a full blood count shows an eosinophil count of 1.5×10^9/l. What is the most likely diagnosis?

☐   A   Eosinophilic granuloma
☐   B   Löeffler's syndrome
☐   C   Pulmonary tuberculosis
☐   D   Sarcoidosis
☐   E   Fibrosing alveolitis

14.11 **A 30-year-old woman underwent bronchoscopy for the investigation of abnormal pulmonary infiltrates seen on a chest X-ray. The biopsy obtained revealed a non-caseating granuloma. Which one of the following statements regarding this condition is true?**

- [ ] A It is a parenchymal lung disease which is often accompanied by pleural effusion
- [ ] B Clubbing of the fingers is an early feature
- [ ] C Jaundice and portal hypertension are the predominant features of hepatic involvement
- [ ] D A positive tuberculin test in chronic cases is suggestive of concomitant tuberculosis
- [ ] E Hypercalcaemia, when manifest, is usually resistant to steroid therapy

14.12 **A 20-year-old woman is admitted with haemoptysis and right-sided pleuritic chest pain. She is short of breath. The chest X-ray is normal. You are considering an urgent ventilation-perfusion ($\dot{V}/\dot{Q}$) scan. Which one of the following statements about $\dot{V}/\dot{Q}$ scans of the lung is true?**

- [ ] A Previous pulmonary embolism does not affect the future scan picture for recurrent pulmonary embolism
- [ ] B A diagnosis of pulmonary embolism cannot be excluded when a scan is reported as normal because of low scan specificity
- [ ] C The scan findings are more informative if the chest X-ray is normal
- [ ] D A diagnosis of pulmonary embolism is more probable when there is a single subsegmental mismatch
- [ ] E These scans help differentiate pulmonary arteriovenous malformation from pulmonary embolism

14.13 A 62-year-old heavy smoker is admitted with increasing shortness of breath, cough and expectoration of green sputum. His notes show that he has had between three and four hospital admissions a year with exacerbations of chronic obstructive pulmonary disease. He is taking steroids, bronchodilators and antibiotics. He improves, and prior to his discharge you are considering long-term home oxygen therapy (LTOT). The presence of which one of the following features is an absolute indication for LTOT?

☐ A Haematocrit ≥55%
☐ B Walking distance of less than 100 yards (90 m) on the level
☐ C Persistent hypoxaemia, PaO_2 <7.3 kPa
☐ D Oxygen saturations (SaO_2) of 90–95%
☐ E FEV_1 between 2 and 3 litres in the first second

14.14 A 63-year-old smoker, who is otherwise healthy, is admitted to hospital with a 3-day history of left-sided chest pain and a cough productive of green sputum. A chest X-ray shows patchy consolidation in the left base. Which of the following is most likely to be responsible for this patient's illness?

☐ A *Streptococcus pneumoniae*
☐ B *Mycoplasma pneumoniae*
☐ C *Staphylococcus aureus*
☐ D *Haemophilus influenzae*
☐ E Viral pneumonia

14.15 A 40-year-old man is referred with a 3-month history of shortness of breath. As you consider the symptom of dyspnoea, which one of the following statements would you consider to be accurate?

☐ A In diaphragmatic paralysis it occurs immediately after lying down
☐ B When it occurs 10 minutes after cessation of exercise, psychogenic hyperventilation may be the cause
☐ C In asthma it is usually worse towards the end of the day
☐ D In pulmonary venous congestion it occurs immediately after sleep
☐ E In hypersensitivity pneumonitis it is worse early in the morning

14.16 A 31-year-old man presents with a cough and expectoration of greenish sputum. He has had recurrent chest infections with progressive shortness of breath since early childhood. A high-resolution computed tomography scan of the chest shows dilated airways in both lower lobes and in the lingula. When seen in cross-section, the dilated airways have a ring-like appearance. Which one of the following disorders is most likely to be the cause of this patient's symptoms?

- ☐ A Asthma
- ☐ B Immotile cilia syndrome (Kartagener's syndrome)
- ☐ C Carcinoma of the bronchus
- ☐ D Mitral valve disease and recurrent pulmonary oedema
- ☐ E Emphysema

14.17 Which one of the following is the main limiting feature of spiral computed tomography scanning for pulmonary embolism?

- ☐ A High level of artefacts due to unavoidable chest movement during respiration
- ☐ B Low sensitivity for detecting pulmonary emboli in main pulmonary arteries
- ☐ C Technical difficulty in passing a catheter into the pulmonary artery
- ☐ D Long scanning time
- ☐ E Low sensitivity for detecting pulmonary emboli in subsegmental pulmonary arteries

14.18 A 50-year-old hospital porter is an in-patient on a surgical ward after a routine keyhole cholecystectomy. He normally smokes 30 cigarettes a day. Five days after the operation he begins to have a high temperature and expectorates green phlegm. A chest X-ray shows consolidation in his right lung. His oxygen saturations are 85% on air. The surgical consultant asks you to assess him. Which one of the following treatments would you choose?

- ☐ A Penicillin + macrolide
- ☐ B Cephalosporin alone
- ☐ C Quinolone alone
- ☐ D Cephalosporin + aminoglycoside
- ☐ E Penicillin + flucloxacillin + macrolide

Answers on pages 267–269

14.19 A 40-year-old woman presents with a 6-month history of dry cough. She is otherwise healthy and takes no regular medications. She has never smoked cigarettes. Physical examination of the chest and heart is normal. Which one of the following steps should be next in the evaluation of this patient's chronic cough?

☐ A   Pulmonary function tests with methacholine challenge
☐ B   High-resolution computed tomography scanning of the chest
☐ C   Chest X-ray
☐ D   Plain X-rays of the nasal sinuses
☐ E   24-hour oesophageal pH monitoring

14.20 A 50-year-old van driver with a normal body mass index is referred to the Sleep Clinic because he keeps failing asleep at the wheel and has had three car crashes. His wife complains that he keeps her awake all night snoring. A sleep study confirms moderate-severity sleep apnoea. Which one of the treatments below would be the most suitable first-line therapy?

☐ A   Long-term oxygen therapy
☐ B   Mandibular advancement splinting
☐ C   Pharyngeal wall surgery
☐ D   Tracheostomy
☐ E   Weight loss

Answers on pages 269–270

Chapter 15

RHEUMATOLOGY AND IMMUNOLOGY

Questions

15.1 A 76-year-old woman with rheumatoid arthritis is referred with a red, painful right eye. Examination reveals an injected conjunctiva with a normal pupil. The visual acuity is normal and no abnormality is detected on examination of the retina. Which of the following is the most likely diagnosis?

☐ A Iritis
☐ B Episcleritis
☐ C Scleritis
☐ D Posterior uveitis
☐ E Macular degeneration

Answers on page 271

15.2 A 70-year-old woman is referred to the Emergency Department with severe unilateral (left-sided) headache. She also claims that she is finding it difficult to chew meat because of pain in her tongue and jaw, although she denies having any problems with swallowing. Her husband says that she is increasingly stiff in the mornings and that her mobility has been in rapid decline, particularly in the last 4 weeks. The full blood count shows a slightly raised white cell count at $12 \times 10^9/l$ and the platelet count is $600 \times 10^9/l$; the erythrocyte sedimentation rate is 110mm/hour. What should your next step in the management be?

- [ ] A   Arrange an urgent computed tomography scan of the brain
- [ ] B   Give 60 mg of prednisolone orally
- [ ] C   Request X-rays of the left temporomandibular joint
- [ ] D   Start intravenous broad-spectrum antibiotic treatment
- [ ] E   Give non-steroidal anti-inflammatory drugs and monitor her progress in a week's time

15.3 Which one of the following statements about the BCG (bacille Calmette–Guérin) vaccine is true?

- [ ] A   The vaccine contains live attenuated human *Mycobacterium tuberculosis*
- [ ] B   It provides immunity against tuberculosis (TB) for 5–10 years
- [ ] C   In the first 4 weeks after vaccination there is a high risk of developing miliary tuberculosis
- [ ] D   In areas where TB is endemic, vaccination is usually offered to children between 10 and 15 years of age
- [ ] E   Subsequent tuberculin tests will be negative

15.4 A 19-year-old student presents with swelling of the face, hands and feet, along with diffuse abdominal pain. He gives a history of recurrent similar episodes since he was 10 years old, at a rate of three to four attacks per year. Each episode would last 2–3 days. The family history reveals that his older brother had similar attacks. Which one of the following tests would be most helpful in establishing the diagnosis?

☐ A   Eosinophil count in the blood
☐ B   Prick (puncture) skin test
☐ C   Radioallergosorbent test (RAST)
☐ D   C1 esterase inhibitor level
☐ E   IgE levels

15.5 A 74-year-old-man is seen for preoperative assessment prior to a right total hip replacement for osteoarthritis which has been scheduled for 8 weeks' time. It was thought that he was fit to have the operation, but the blood tests show raised immunoglobulins and the immune electrophoresis has identified a monoclonal band of the IgG type at 2.5 g/dl. On reviewing his old records, a similar immunoglobulin abnormality was noted a year ago. Further tests, however, reveal no lytic bone lesions on skeletal survey and no Bence Jones proteinuria. What is the most likely underlying disease?

☐ A   Carcinoma of the prostate
☐ B   Multiple myeloma
☐ C   Rheumatoid arthritis
☐ D   Monoclonal gammopathy of undetermined significance (MGUS)
☐ E   Waldenström's macroglobulinaemia

Answers on pages 271–272

15.6   **Which one of the following statements about inflammatory indicators is true?**

☐   A   The erythrocyte sedimentation rate (ESR) is elevated in hypoalbuminaemia

☐   B   The C-reactive protein (CRP) level is generally elevated in primary Sjögren's syndrome

☐   C   A rise in plasma viscosity is primarily due to an increase in the haematocrit

☐   D   The plasma viscosity test is generally less specific and less sensitive than the ESR

☐   E   CRP is produced by the subthalamic nucleus in the brain

15.7   **You are investigating a patient with glomerulonephritis. A renal biopsy tissue specimen was reported as, 'There are no immune deposits on immunohistochemical analysis.' This is characteristic of which one of the following renal disorders?**

☐   A   Systemic lupus erythematosus (SLE)

☐   B   Henoch–Schönlein nephritis

☐   C   Goodpasture's syndrome

☐   D   Wegener's granulomatosis

☐   E   Buerger's disease

15.8   **Which one of the following statements about the immune system is true?**

☐   A   Class II major histocompatibility complex (MHC) antigens are present on virtually all human cell types

☐   B   The liver clears IgM-sensitised erythrocytes

☐   C   Interleukin 2 (IL-2) is produced exclusively by T lymphocytes

☐   D   The active complement component, C5a stimulates the activation of the alternative complement pathway

☐   E   Erythrocyte destruction in paroxysmal nocturnal haemoglobinuria takes place within the liver

15.9 A 66-year-old woman presents with a vasculitic skin rash on her legs. She was recently investigated for recurrent joint swelling and was noted to have significant proteinuria. Essential mixed cryoglobulinaemia (EMC) is considered. Which one of the following is one of the main features associated with this disorder?

- [ ] A Bence Jones protein in the urine
- [ ] B Cold agglutinins in the blood
- [ ] C Osteolytic bone lesions
- [ ] D Cold intolerance
- [ ] E Hepatitis C infection

15.10 A 23-year-old cashier is referred with a history of recurrent attacks of pain and numbness in the fingers of both hands on exposure to cold. She also describes blanching and blue discoloration of the fingers during these attacks. Which one of the following statements best describes primary Raynaud's phenomenon?

- [ ] A It is more common in middle-aged women
- [ ] B Digital gangrene is a frequent complication
- [ ] C The antinuclear antibody is positive in 70% of cases
- [ ] D Nail-fold capillaroscopy shows dilated vessels
- [ ] E The fingers are symmetrically involved during an attack

15.11 Which one of the following types of arthritis is the most common type of psoriatic arthropathy?

- [ ] A Distal interphalangeal (DIP) joint disease
- [ ] B Arthritis mutilans
- [ ] C Peripheral symmetrical polyarthropathy
- [ ] D Peripheral asymmetrical oligoarthropathy
- [ ] E Psoriatic spondylitis

15.12 Which one of the following would be characteristic of the laboratory findings in a patient with the antiphospholipid syndrome?

☐　A　Low C3 and C4 concentrations
☐　B　Positive anticardiolipin antibodies
☐　C　Prolonged INR
☐　D　Elevated low-density lipoprotein (LDL)
☐　E　Thrombocytosis

15.13 A 47-year-old teacher presents with Raynaud's phenomenon. She has multiple necrotic ulcers at the tips of the middle and ring fingers. Examination also shows sclerodactyly and facial telangiectasia. Which one of the following clinical findings is most characteristic of this disorder?

☐　A　Pulmonary hypertension is generally due to recurrent pulmonary embolism
☐　B　The erythrocyte sedimentation rate (ESR) is usually elevated with active disease
☐　C　Alveolar-cell carcinoma of the lung is a recognised complication
☐　D　Cutaneous involvement is invariably present in all forms of the disease
☐　E　Skin thickening characteristically occurs distal to the metacarpophalangeal (MCP) joints

15.14 A 22-year-old shop assistant presents with fever, rigors and severe joint pain and swelling. An intravenous antibiotic is given after a sample of synovial fluid is obtained. Which one of the following features is most suggestive of gonococcal arthritis?

☐　A　Monoarthritis at the outset of the disease
☐　B　Tenosynovitis
☐　C　Episcleritis
☐　D　Cloudy synovial fluid with a white cell count of less than 800/mm³
☐　E　Fever

15.15 A 36-year-old woman with an 8-month history of Raynaud's phenomenon presents to the Emergency Department with recent-onset precordial chest pain. Physical examination reveals a pericardial friction rub and her creatine kinase is elevated five times above the upper normal limit, but the MB (myocardial-bound) isoenzyme is negative. The immunology profile reveals a positive antinuclear antibody (ANA) test at 1 in 640, with a speckled staining pattern. Which of the following is the most appropriate immunological test to organise at this stage?

☐   A   Anti-double-stranded DNA (anti-dsDNA)
☐   B   Antiribonucleoprotein (anti-RNP) antibody
☐   C   Anticentromere antibody
☐   D   Rheumatoid factor
☐   E   Anti-neutrophil cytoplasmic antibody (ANCA)

15.16 An otherwise healthy 48-year-old man presents with an acutely painful right knee. Aspiration and examination of the synovial fluid is positive for calcium pyrophosphate dihydrate (CPPD). Which one of the following tests should be performed to identify a possible underlying cause?

☐   A   Erythrocyte sedimentation rate
☐   B   Serum cortisol
☐   C   Serum ferritin
☐   D   Full blood count
☐   E   Blood culture

15.17 A 70-year-old woman with a 20-year history of rheumatoid arthritis, who is maintained on D-penicillamine (375 mg), presents with a 2-week history of increasing difficulty in climbing stairs. Her husband adds that he has had to wash her hair in the last 4 days. On examination, the neck and shoulder movements are very restricted. Neurological assessment reveals grade 3/5 weakness in both upper and lower limb muscle groups; intact touch and pinprick sensation; normal tendon reflexes; and a positive Babinski sign bilaterally. What is the most probable cause of her recent weakness?

- [ ] A Spinal cord compression due to cervical myelopathy from atlanto-axial subluxation
- [ ] B D-penicillamine-induced myasthenia gravis
- [ ] C Peripheral neuropathy associated with the rheumatoid arthritis
- [ ] D Parasagittal cerebral rheumatoid nodule
- [ ] E Generalised weakness due to disuse muscle atrophy secondary to chronic arthritis

15.18 A 32-year-old man is referred with bouts of low back pain which have been waking him at night for about 6 months. The pain is localised to the lower lumbar region and the buttock. He has had to change his job from working in a warehouse, doing heavy lifting, to a clerical position. He finds that he has to wake himself an hour or two earlier to loosen up so that he can get to work in the morning on time. His past medical history reveals that he had a malignant skin melanoma surgically removed 2 years ago. What is the most probable diagnosis in this case?

- [ ] A Intervertebral disc prolapse and sciatica
- [ ] B Spinal canal stenosis
- [ ] C Ankylosing spondylitis
- [ ] D Melanoma recurrence and spread to vertebrae
- [ ] E Osteomyelitis of the lower lumbar vertebrae

15.19 A 60-year-old woman with dry mouth and dry eyes is found to have a positive Schirmer's test and anti-Ro antibodies. Which one of the following tumours is most likely to complicate this disease?

☐   A   Lymphoma
☐   B   Renal cell carcinoma
☐   C   Hepatoma
☐   D   Thyroid follicular carcinoma
☐   E   Parotid adenoma

15.20 A 50-year-old man is referred with a 2-week history of fever, arthralgia and weight loss. During his hospital stay he develops epigastric pain and notices difficulty in dorsiflexing his left great toe. His blood pressure is 160/95 mmHg. Laboratory studies reveal: haemoglobin 10 g/dl, mean corpuscular volume 98 fl, erythrocyte sedimentation rate 100 mm/hour, and a polymorphonuclear leucocytosis. The chest X-ray is clear. Which one of the following is the most likely diagnosis?

☐   A   Wegener's granulomatosis
☐   B   Systemic lupus erythematosus
☐   C   Polyarteritis nodosa
☐   D   Polymyalgia rheumatica
☐   E   Churg–Strauss syndrome

15.21 A 54-year-old woman who is experiencing increasing generalised pain and discomfort in her neck, shoulders, lower back, hips and knees, is referred for further assessment. She admits to having had these symptoms for 4 years. There is no history of joint swelling, skin rash or Raynaud's phenomenon. She also complains of marked fatigue and tiredness. She gave up her long-term job as a superstore manager 6 months ago. Review of systems reveals increasing urinary urgency and recurrent headaches. On examination, there is no significant abnormality apart from multiple tender spots over the spine and limbs. Blood tests reveal a white cell count of $4 \times 10^9/l$ and a platelet count of $167 \times 10^9/l$; the erythrocyte sedimentation rate is 20 mm/hour. The rheumatoid factor is negative and the ANA test comes back positive at 1 in 40. The creatine kinase and thyroid function tests are within normal limits. Which one of the following is the most probable diagnosis?

- [ ] A Systemic lupus erythematosus
- [ ] B Fibromyalgia syndrome
- [ ] C Chronic fatigue syndrome
- [ ] D Hypothyroidism
- [ ] E Depression

15.22 Which one of the following statements about neuropathic (Charcot) joints is true?

- [ ] A Diabetes mellitus is the most common cause
- [ ] B In children they usually complicate poliomyelitis
- [ ] C The joint often looks normal on clinical examination
- [ ] D Syringomyelia predominantly affects the knees
- [ ] E Joint replacement is the treatment of choice

15.23 A 55-year-old woman is referred because of recent-onset joint pain and prolonged morning stiffness. She is noted to have a necrotic skin rash on both lower limbs. Blood tests show: urea 27 mmol/l, creatinine 360 μmol/l; the ANCA is strongly positive. Which one of the following is the most likely diagnosis?

- ☐ A   Systemic lupus erythematosus
- ☐ B   Takayasu's disease
- ☐ C   Giant-cell arteritis
- ☐ D   Microscopic polyangiitis
- ☐ E   Goodpasture's syndrome

15.24 Which one of the following is often associated with low uric acid levels?

- ☐ A   Thiazide diuretic therapy
- ☐ B   Alcoholism
- ☐ C   Polycythaemia rubra vera
- ☐ D   Eclampsia of pregnancy
- ☐ E   Psoriasis

15.25 A 47-year-old woman presents with an inability to raise her arms above her shoulders. Over the past few weeks she has also been having difficulty swallowing food. On examination, there is muscle wasting and the muscles are tender, with reduced tendon reflexes. Her serum creatine kinase is elevated. What is the most likely diagnosis?

- ☐ A   Polymyalgia rheumatica
- ☐ B   Polymyositis
- ☐ C   Hypocalcaemia
- ☐ D   Painful arc syndrome
- ☐ E   Frozen shoulder

Chapter 16
STATISTICS
Questions

16.1 Which one of the following statements concerning the distribution curve is accurate?

☐ A The mode is the sum of all the scores divided by the number of scores

☐ B The mean is a good measure of central tendency

☐ C The mean is higher than the median in a positively skewed distribution

☐ D When there is an even number of numbers, the mode is the mean of the two middle numbers

☐ E In any given distribution there is only one mode

6.2 In a study, the odds of a disease occurring in the group of subjects who smoke are 0.25. Which one of the following is therefore true?

☐ A Smoking causes the disease

☐ B For every four people who smoke, one has the disease

☐ C For every five people who smoke, one has the disease

☐ D The disease occurs four times more often in those who smoke

☐ E A larger sample is needed

Answers on page 284–285

16.3   A study is designed to assess the safety of recombinant human erythropoietin (rhEPO) when used in premature infants of less than 33 weeks' gestation to reduce postnatal haemoglobin decline. Out of 31 infants given the treatment, none suffered serious side-effects. Which one of the conclusions listed below can be reached from this study?

- ☐ A   rhEPO is safe
- ☐ B   rhEPO is safe when used in the dosages used in this study
- ☐ C   Nothing conclusive can be claimed; a larger study is required
- ☐ D   rhEPO does not cause serious side-effects when used in moderate doses
- ☐ E   Premature infants of less than 33 weeks' gestation can safely be given rhEPO

16.4   In a small double-blind study of pain following dental surgery, patients are randomly allocated to receive either an analgesic tablet or a matching placebo tablet 1 hour preoperatively. All patients were asked to rate their pain 4 hours after surgery using the following scale: 0 = none, 1 = mild, 2 = moderate, 3 = severe. Which one of the following is the best statistical test for analysing the results of this study?

- ☐ A   Chi-square test
- ☐ B   One-way analysis of variance
- ☐ C   Mann–Whitney U-test
- ☐ D   Fisher's exact test
- ☐ E   Unpaired Student's t-test

16.5 **In a study of 100 normal men aged 40–49 years, the FEV$_1$ levels were found to be approximately normally distributed, with a mean value of 3.50 litres. The 95% confidence limits for the mean were calculated as 3.34–3.66 litres. Which of the following statements is most accurate?**

◻ A   5% of subjects will have FEV$_1$ levels less than 3.34 litres

◻ B   2.5% of subjects will have FEV$_1$ levels less than 3.34 litres

◻ C   If another group of normal men of the same age was studied, the sample mean FEV$_1$ would have a 95% chance of being between 3.34 litres and 3.66 litres

◻ D   The 95% confidence limits can be used to screen subjects for abnormal respiratory function

◻ E   The range of values, 3.34–3.66 litres, excludes the population mean with a probability of 0.05

Answers on pages 285–286   131

Answers and Teaching Notes

Chapter 1

BASIC SCIENCES

Answers

1.1　**A:　It packages molecules into vesicles that can be transported out of a cell**

The Golgi apparatus consists of stacks of membrane-covered sacs that package and move proteins to the outside of the cell. The mitochondria are the enzyme-rich organelles that produce most of the ATP energy. The centriole is involved in cell division. The ribosome contains ribonucleic acid molecules and enzymes that are required for manufacturing proteins. Phagocytosis is not a function of the Golgi apparatus.

1.2　**A:　Programmed cell death**

Apoptosis is defined as 'programmed cell death'. This occurs in individual cells, with no associated inflammatory reaction, in contrast to cell necrosis. It is a crucial process in embryogenesis, when tissue building, replacement and moulding are at their peak. Unopposed apoptosis with progressive destruction of specific groups of nerve cells is thought to be one of the processes that ultimately leads to Alzheimer's disease. On the other hand, inhibition of apoptosis, with prolonged cell survival, may have a determinant role in the induction of autoimmunity (prolonging immunocompetent cell survival). Similarly, in lung cancer, genetic abnormalities such as mutation of the oncogene *TP53* can lead to loss of tumour suppression function, inhibition of apoptosis and increased cellular proliferation. Recent investigation of bone marrow myeloid progenitor cells in myelodysplasia and cyclic neutropenia suggests that intramedullary apoptosis is a central feature regulating cell loss in this disorder. The pathogenesis of ischaemic heart disease involves cell death due to necrosis and this is associated with a local inflammatory reaction. Proptosis is forward movement of the eyeball. Tenosynovitis is inflammation of the tendon sheath.

1.3   E: Transforming growth factor β (TGF-β) inhibits the production of other cytokines

Cytokines are hormone-like proteins that enable the immune cells to communicate. They play an important role in initiation, perpetuation and subsequent down-regulation of the immune response. They are produced by immune system cells and also by non-immune system cells such as fibroblasts and endothelial cells. Interleukin 6 (IL-6) enhances the production of the acute-phase reactant proteins in the liver but does not enhance the production of albumin, which is not an acute-phase reactant. IL-2, produced by T cells, increases expression of its own receptor on T cells and markedly enhances T-cell proliferation. Distinct subsets of helper T cells have been identified by virtue of the cytokines that they produce: T_H1 cells regulate delayed-type hypersensitivity reactions and T_H2 cells mediate allergic and antibody responses.

1.4   D: The spermatozoon concentration may be temporarily suppressed by fever

Normal ejaculate volume ranges from 2 ml to 6 ml. The normal range of spermatozoon concentration is 20–200 million per ml and up to 20% are morphologically abnormal. More than 60% of spermatozoa examined within 1 hour after ejaculation are motile. In any individual, sperm counts exhibit extreme variability and are often temporarily suppressed by factors such as fever. In a human it takes approximately 3 months for complete maturation of a spermatozoon. Semen is produced in the testes and stored in the seminal vesicles. Sildenafil (Viagra®) has been licensed for the treatment of impotence. It causes vasodilatation of the corpora cavernosa blood vessels and so increases the blood flow and maintains erection in the penis. Viagra® has no direct effect on sperm count or fertility.

1.5   E: Angiotensin II

Renin is a glycoprotein of 274 amino acids and is produced in the juxtaglomerular cells of the afferent renal arteriole. It converts angiotensinogen to angiotensin I. It is stimulated by a lowering of the blood pressure. Angiotensin II and vasopressin inhibit renin release.

1.6   B: Abductor pollicis brevis

The median nerve supplies the following structures in the hand:

- abductor pollicis brevis, flexor pollicis brevis, opponens pollicis
- lateral two lumbricals
- the skin of the lateral three and half fingers.

The ulnar nerve supplies all the interossei and the rest of the hand muscles.

1.7   C: It increases the concentrations of circulating factor VIII and von Willebrand factor

Arginine vasopressin (AVP; antidiuretic hormone, ADH) is synthesised in the supraoptic and paraventricular nuclei of the hypothalamus. V2 receptors mediate its antidiuretic effect. It makes the distal convoluted tubules more permeable to hypotonic fluid. It stimulates ACTH release and increases concentrations of circulating factor VIII and von Willebrand factor. By stimulating V1 receptors it causes vasoconstriction of splanchnic, renal and coronary vessels, and promotes glycogenolysis.

1.8   B: Osteoclasts

Osteopetrosis is an inherited disorder characterised by increased bone density. In severe forms the bone marrow cavity may be obliterated. The primary underlying defect in all types of osteopetrosis is failure of the osteoclasts to reabsorb bone. This results in thickened sclerotic bones. Radiological features are usually diagnostic. Bones may be uniformly sclerotic.

1.9   D: There is increased renal excretion of bicarbonate

Physiological acclimatisation starts at about 7000 feet (2100 m).
The partial pressure of atmospheric oxygen reduces with altitude.
Pulmonary ventilation and perfusion increase, plasma volume
decreases and renal excretion of bicarbonate increases. These
changes serve to maintain the arterial oxygen tension. Erythrocyte
production increases and the haemoglobin concentration and
haematocrit increase. Above 1400 feet, the heart rate, cardiac
output and pulmonary artery pressure increase. Alveolar
hypoventilation, hypoxia and cyanosis are features of chronic
mountain sickness when the physiological response of
acclimatisation is no longer maintained.

1.10   B: Urine osmolality of 120 mosmol/kg

The main features (diagnostic criteria) of SIADH consist of
hyponatraemia and hypotonicity (<280 mosmol/kg), the absence
of fluid volume depletion, inappropriately high urinary osmolality
(>100 mosmol/kg), and increased urinary sodium excretion
(>40 mmol/l) while on a normal salt and water intake, and the
absence of thyroid, adrenal, pituitary or renal dysfunction.
Although a low serum potassium concentration and a normal
urine output are consistent with the diagnosis of SIADH, they are
not exclusive to SIADH (neither their presence nor their absence
would confirm or exclude this diagnosis).

1.11   C: Stroke volume

During exercise, increased oxygen consumption and increased
venous return to the heart result in an increase in cardiac output
and an increase in blood flow to both skeletal muscle and the
coronary circulation, when oxygen utilisation is greatest. The
increase in cardiac output is due to an increase in both heart rate
and stroke volume. The systemic arterial pressure also increases in
response to the increase in cardiac output. However, the fall in
total peripheral resistance, which is caused by dilatation of the
blood vessels within the exercising muscles, results in a decrease
in the diastolic blood pressure. The pulmonary vessels undergo
passive dilatation as more blood flows into the pulmonary
circulation. As a result, pulmonary vascular resistance decreases.

The decrease in venous compliance, caused by sympathetic stimulation, helps to maintain ventricular filling during diastole.

1.12   A: In heart failure it is associated with a poor prognosis

In heart failure, reduced cardiac output will cause reduced renal blood flow, increase of aldosterone secretion and sympathetic activity, which result in salt and water retention by the kidneys. ADH is increased in heart failure, causing further limitation of free water excretion. Together with the increased thirst in patients with advanced heart failure, this leads to a hyponatraemic state that is a particularly ominous prognostic sign. Hyponatraemia in liver disease is typically due to a combination of reduced renal clearance of free water and administration of excessive free water. Mineralocorticoid deficiency causes increased urinary clearance of sodium with volume contraction and increased ADH, which reduces free water excretion. The clinical features of hyponatraemia generally manifest when the serum sodium concentration falls to 120 mmol/l or less. Paraproteinaemia causes false hyponatraemia (with normal osmolarity) due to displacement of more fluid in the serum, which gives falsely low sodium readings.

1.13   A: $\dot{V}/\dot{Q}$ ratio

The alveoli at the apex of the lung are larger than those at the base, so they are less compliant. Because of the reduced compliance, less inspired gas goes to the apex than to the base. Also, because the apex is above heart level, less blood flows through the apex than through the base. However, the reduction in air flow is less than the reduction in blood flow, so that the $\dot{V}/\dot{Q}$ ratio at the top of the lung is greater than it is at the bottom. The increased $\dot{V}/\dot{Q}$ ratio at the apex makes the $Pa\text{CO}_2$ lower and the $Pa\text{O}_2$ higher at the apex than they are at the base.

1.14   B: Dopamine

The pathogenesis of Parkinson's disease is multifactorial, characterised by progressive death of heterogeneous populations of neurones, particularly in the substantia nigra, and resulting in a regional loss of the neurotransmitter dopamine. A 60–70% loss of neurones occurs prior to the emergence of symptoms.

1.15   B: Aschoff nodules in rheumatic fever

A 'pathognomonic' symptom or sign is a symptom or sign unique to a particular disease. The presence of such a symptom or sign allows positive diagnosis of the disease. Although the histological diagnosis of Hodgkin's disease requires the presence of Reed–Sternberg cells, these cells are not pathognomonic of the disease and have been described in infectious mononucleosis, other viral infections, and malignancies. Aschoff nodules, considered pathognomonic of rheumatic fever, consist of a central area of fibrinoid surrounded by lymphocytes, plasma cells, and large basophilic cells, some of which are multinucleated. Charcot–Leyden crystals (CLCs) have been found in many conditions associated with eosinophilia. Crystals of CLC protein in body fluids and secretions have long been considered a hallmark of eosinophil-associated allergic inflammatory diseases such as asthma, allergic rhinitis and atopic dermatitis. Alcoholic hyaline (Mallory body) is not specific for alcoholic liver disease because it has been detected in the livers of patients with Wilson's disease, primary biliary cirrhosis, hepatic carcinoma and also following jejuno-ileal bypass. The presence of non-caseating granuloma should not be construed as diagnostic of sarcoidosis until a thorough investigation of other causes of granulomatous inflammation has been conducted.

1.16   B: Exercise

Growth hormone (GH) is synthesised, stored, and secreted by the endocrine cells of the anterior pituitary. Its release is stimulated by growth hormone-releasing hormone and inhibited by somatostatin. Numerous factors stimulate GH release, including hypoglycaemia (eg insulin administration), moderate to severe exercise, stress due to emotional disturbances, illness, fever, and dopamine agonists such as bromocriptine.

1.17   E: The nucleus

Receptors for steroid and thyroid hormones are located inside the target cell nucleus, and function as 'ligand-dependent transcription factors'. That is to say, the hormone–receptor complex binds to promoter regions of responsive genes and stimulates or sometimes inhibits transcription from those genes. Protein and peptide hormones, catecholamines and prostaglandins find their receptors on the plasma membrane of target cells. Binding of hormone to receptor initiates a series of events which leads to generation of so-called 'second messengers' within the cell (the hormone is the first messenger). The second messengers (cyclic AMP, protein kinase, calcium and/or phospho-inositides and cyclic GMP) then trigger a series of molecular interactions that alter the physiological state of the cell. Another term used to describe this entire process is 'signal transduction'.

1.18   C: It has a lower glucose concentration than plasma

Cerebrospinal fluid (CSF) is formed primarily in the choroid plexus by an active secretory process. It circulates in the subarachnoid space, between the dura mater and the pia mater, and is absorbed into the circulation via the arachnoid villi. The epidural space, which lies outside the dura mater, may be used clinically for instillation of anaesthetics. CSF protein and glucose concentrations are much lower than those in the plasma.

1.19   C: Hyponatraemia

Aldosterone is a mineralocorticoid secreted by the zona glomerulosa layer of the adrenal gland. Its main action is on the kidneys, causing sodium and water retention. Renin and angiotensin II stimulate aldosterone production. An increased serum potassium level stimulates its release, and a reduced potassium level inhibits its release; a change of as little as 0.1 mmol/l will affect aldosterone secretion independently of sodium or angiotensin II. ACTH has a transient stimulatory effect and chronic ACTH deficiency rarely blunts aldosterone production. Hyponatraemia reduces and hypernatraemia increases aldosterone release: these influences are probably mediated through the effect of renin. Dopamine agonists (eg bromocriptine) inhibit aldosterone secretion while dopamine antagonists stimulate its release.

1.20   B: It promotes inflammation

The main sources of TNF are the activated cells of the monocyte phagocytic system and, to a lesser extent, antigen-stimulated T cells, natural killer (NK) cells and activated mast cells. TNF plays a central role in the immune system and appears to be particularly critical for innate immunity. It is an important mediator of local inflammation and appears to be vital in keeping infections localised. TNF causes local activation of vascular endothelium, release of nitric oxide with vasodilatation, increased vascular permeability, increased expression of adhesion molecules on the endothelium of blood vessels, and increased expression of class II major histocompatibility (MHC) molecules. The result is recruitment of inflammatory cells, immunoglobulins and complement. It promotes angiogenesis.

TNF plays a central role in the pathological inflammatory response associated with rheumatoid arthritis. Evidence to support this statement includes the finding of excessively high TNF levels in the serum; the correlation between an abundance of macrophage products (TNF, interleukins 1, 6, and 8) in the synovial tissue and fluid with the severity and activity of disease; and, most important, the consistent improvement in disease activity, both symptomatically and radiographically, when therapy is directed against TNF. Anti-TNF-α therapies reduce inflammation and inhibit the progression of rheumatoid arthritis. Many studies have confirmed that this type of therapy is effective in various inflammatory conditions and that the risk of solid or haematological malignancy is not significantly higher than in placebo groups.

1.21   C: Cutaneous

Hypoxia activates chemoreceptors, causing a sympathetic vasoconstrictor response in the skin, skeletal muscle and splanchnic beds. In contrast, in the presence of hypoxia the coronary, cerebral and renovascular beds undergo vasodilatation, thus permitting the redistribution of blood to the vital organs, with their higher oxygen demands.

1.22   E: Hiccup is caused by spasmodic contraction of the diaphragm

The diaphragm is composed of skeletal muscle and a central tendon. When the muscle contracts, the diaphragm descends. Paradoxical upward movement of the diaphragm and inward movement of the abdominal wall during inspiration occur when there is bilateral paralysis of the diaphragm. Normally, the right dome of the diaphragm is higher than the left one. The diaphragm is higher on the paralysed side on X-ray examination. Each hemidiaphragm is supplied by the corresponding phrenic nerve. Hiccup is believed to be due to mechanical or metabolic irritation of the phrenic nerve, leading to spasmodic contraction of the diaphragm.

1.23   B: Squamous

Hypercalcaemia is the most common metabolic abnormality associated with cancer. Parathyroid hormone-related peptide (PTHrP) has emerged as the main mediator of hypercalcaemia, not only in squamous-cell tumours (eg of lung, skin, head and neck, cervix, vulva), but also in breast, renal, or ovarian carcinomas, pancreatic islet cell tumours, phaeochromocytomas and haematological malignancies such as leukaemias, lymphomas and multiple myeloma.

In general, PTHrP is a humoral factor that circulates in the bloodstream and is transported to bone, where it stimulates bone resorption through the PTH/PTHrP receptor. However, it may also be produced locally by tumour cells that have metastasised to bone, often in conjunction with cytokines such as interleukin 6 (IL-6). PTHrP, IL-6 and other factors synergistically stimulate osteoclast-mediated bone resorption, as well as the production by osteoclasts of tumour growth factors such as transforming growth factor β (TGF-β). TGF-β in turn stimulates further PTHrP production, thus setting in motion and amplifying an ineluctable process of tumour growth and hypercalcaemia. Therefore, by inhibiting osteoclasts, bisphosphonates such as pamidronate not only decrease hypercalcaemia and skeletal morbidity, but also tumour burden. One of the most exciting findings in this field in recent years is the fact that bisphosphonates may actually improve quality of life and prolong survival in patients with breast cancer and multiple myeloma.

Tumour cell type	Hormone
Neuroendocrine	Adrenocorticotrophic hormone (ACTH)
	Arginine vasopressin (AVP)/Antidiuretic hormone (ADP)
	Corticotrophin-releasing factor (CRF)
	Growth hormone-releasing factor (GHRH)
	Somatostatin
	Calcitonin
Squamous	Parathyroid hormone-related peptide (PTHrP)
Large cell	Human chorionic gonadotrophin (hCG)
Mesenchymal	Insulin-like growth factor II (IGF-II)
	Phosphaturic factor

1.24 D: Homozygous C2 deficiency is associated with systemic lupus erythematosus (SLE)

Only IgG and IgM can activate the classical pathway, as other antibody classes are not capable of binding C1 complement. In hereditary angio-oedema the cause is C1INH (C1 esterase inhibitor) deficiency and not C1 complement deficiency. C1, C2 and C4 are typically normal when the alternative pathway is activated. Inherited deficiency of C1q, C2 and C4 is associated with a high incidence of autoimmune diseases (SLE, vasculitis) while deficiency of complement C5, C6, C7 and C8 is associated with selective propensity for developing disseminated *Neisseria* infection. Renal disease in scleroderma resembles the nephropathy of malignant hypertension; hypocomplementaemia is not a feature of this disorder.

1.25 C: The vast majority of obese individuals have markedly elevated plasma leptin concentrations

The discovery of leptin continued the hormonal link between the adipocyte and the brain. Leptin is mainly secreted by the adipocyte, circulates in part while linked to binding proteins, and acts in specific regions of the brain (hypothalamus) to regulate appetite and energy balance. Daily injections of leptin decreased appetite and body weight in both *ob/ob* mice and wild-type mice and increased energy expenditure in lean newborn Zucker rats. Leptin deficiency caused genetic obesity in *ob/ob* mice as well as in a recently described family kindred. The vast majority of obese individuals have markedly elevated plasma leptin concentrations when compared with lean individuals. In fact, plasma leptin concentrations strongly correlate with the percentage of body fat and leptin levels are reduced in obese subjects who lose weight. A higher set point of the cerebral adipostat present in obese individuals may be the result of a relative or absolute insensitivity to leptin. This has led to the notion that 'leptin resistance' underlies most cases of obesity.

1.26 C: It reduces urinary calcium excretion, which reduces the risk of kidney stones

Epidemiological and clinical studies have shown that potassium intake has an important role in regulating blood pressure in both the general population and individuals with high blood pressure. High potassium intake reduces blood pressure in both hypertensive and normotensive individuals. It may have other beneficial effects which are independent of its effect on blood pressure, such as reducing the risk of stroke and preventing the development of renal vascular, glomerular and tubular damage. Increasing potassium intake reduces calcium excretion and causes a positive calcium balance that may be associated in the longer term with a higher bone mass. A reduction in calcium excretion is associated with reduced risk of kidney stones. Increasing serum potassium concentrations reduces the risk of ventricular arrhythmias in patients with ischaemic heart disease, heart failure and left ventricular hypertrophy. High potassium intake has no effect on blood cholesterol levels.

1.27 B: 1500 mg/day of calcium, 400–800 units/day of vitamin D

Adequate calcium and vitamin D intake should be part of both the prevention and the treatment of osteoporosis. Dietary intake of calcium should be 800–1000 mg/day in childhood through to early adulthood, 1000–1200 mg/day in the middle years, and 1500 mg/day in the elderly. If osteoporosis is established, the treatment includes 1500 mg/day of calcium and 400–800 units/ day of vitamin D.

1.28   E: Levels are typically normal in DiGeorge syndrome

IgG is the only antibody that crosses the placenta. IgM has the highest molecular weight, but IgG has the highest concentration in plasma. All immunoglobulins are synthesised by lymphocytes. DiGeorge syndrome is characterised by dysmorphogenesis of the third and the fourth pharyngeal pouches, leading to hypoplasia or aplasia of the thymus and the parathyroid gland. It manifests as hypocalcaemic fits in the neonate, a low T lymphocyte cell count, a high B lymphocyte cell count and, typically, normal immunoglobulin levels.

1.29   B: Antiplatelet

COX-2 inhibition is responsible for the analgesic and the anti-inflammatory effects of celecoxib and other COX-2 inhibitors (known as 'coxibs') which appear indistinguishable from those of several standard non-steroidal anti-inflammatory drugs (NSAIDs), which predominantly inhibit COX-1. The renal effects of coxibs are similar to those of non-selective traditional NSAIDs. They cause sodium and water retention; both are associated with increased incidence of peripheral oedema and worsening of pre-existing hypertension. Coxibs can cause bronchospasm and, rarely, angio-oedema, as with other NSAIDs. Unlike older, non-selective COX inhibitors, COX-2 inhibitors do not decrease the production of thromboxane in platelets and therefore do not inhibit platelet aggregation or increase bleeding time. As normal platelet function is preserved in patients on selective COX-2 inhibitors, patients requiring cardioprotective antiplatelet therapy should continue low-dose aspirin.

1.30   A: 345 mosmol/kg

Plasma osmolality, a major determinant of total body water homeostasis, is measured by the number of solute particles present in 1 kg of plasma. It is calculated in mmol per litre, using this formula: $2 \times [Na^+] + [urea] + [glucose]$.

Chapter 2

CARDIOLOGY

Answers

2.1 A: Right coronary artery

ST-segment elevation in leads II, III, and aVF usually indicates blockage in the artery supplying the inferior wall of the left ventricle. The infarction often stems from an occlusion of the distal portion of the right coronary artery.

2.2 A: Atrial septal defect (ASD)

Atrial septal defect (ASD) causes wide splitting of the second heart sound. This is due to increased flow through the pulmonary artery, which causes delay in the pulmonary component of the second heart sound. The other answer stems in the question are associated with paradoxical splitting of the second heart sound, which could be due to:

* late A2 (aortic component of the second heart sound), which occurs in LBBB, aortic stenosis and PDA
* early P2 (pulmonary component of the second heart sound), which occurs in type B WPW syndrome.

2.3 A: The coarctation is proximal to the origin of the left subclavian artery if the right arm blood pressure is significantly higher than that in the left arm

The commonest site of discrete obstruction of the aortic lumen is just distal to the origin of the left subclavian artery. If the systolic arterial pressure in the right arm is higher than that in the left arm by more than 30 mmHg, the left subclavian is involved in the coarctation. The systolic arterial pressure in the arms exceeds that in the leg. A continuous murmur over the thoracic spine usually originates from a small, tight coarctation (<2 mm). Other cardiac malformations are frequent, the commonest being a bicuspid aortic valve. Notching of the inferior border of the ribs by collateral vessels is common and usually manifest in adults and in older children. Patients with coarctation are at high risk of subacute bacterial endocarditis and should be strongly advised about antibiotic prophylaxis.

2.4   C: Echocardiogram is diagnostic in most cases

Atrial myxoma is a benign tumour of the heart. Approximately 75% originate in the left atrium. The clinical features are characterised by a triad of embolism, intracardiac obstruction and constitutional symptoms. The clinical signs can mimic mitral stenosis and the murmur may vary with body position. Fragments of tumour break off easily but do not grow in peripheral sites. Recurrence is very rare after complete and careful removal of the tumour.

2.5   C: If *Streptococcus bovis* endocarditis is diagnosed, a thorough investigation of the colon is indicated

Streptococcus bovis endocarditis is often associated with colonic carcinomas and polyps. The most common cause of negative blood cultures in a patient with infective endocarditis is prior antimicrobial therapy. Early prosthetic valve endocarditis occurs within 60 days of valve placement. *Staphylococcus epidermidis* is the leading cause of early valve endocarditis. Prophylaxis for endocarditis is probably not required to cover for cardiac catheterisation, insertion of a pacemaker, bronchoscopy, endoscopy, normal vaginal delivery or dilation and curettage. Cystoscopy is one of the procedures that does require antibiotic prophylaxis, however.

2.6   E: Digoxin therapy

Digoxin's effect is characterised by a short QT interval. Prolonged QT interval is usually associated with the use of class I antiarrhythmic drugs (quinidine, procainamide) and other drugs like phenytoin and tricyclic antidepressants. Electrolyte imbalance, especially hypokalaemia and hypomagnesaemia, can cause a prolonged QT interval. Other causes of prolonged QT interval include acute myocardial infarction, myocarditis, hypothermia and amiodarone therapy.

2.7   A: *Staphylococcus aureus* is the most frequent causative agent

Staphylococcus aureus alone accounts for 50–70% of cases. Large vegetations are typical. It can infect a normal heart valve. Metastatic abscesses are more common in the acute form of the disease. Abscesses in the fibrocardiac skeleton tissue or in the myocardium are also much more likely to be found in acute bacterial endocarditis than in subacute bacterial endocarditis. They might cause conduction defects if they are adjacent to the fibres of the conduction system.

2.8   C: Measurement of the pulmonary artery wedge pressure

The adult respiratory distress syndrome (ARDS) is a clinical triad of hypoxaemia, diffuse lung infiltrates and reduced lung compliance which is not attributable to congestive cardiac failure. This has been reported as a complication of apparently unrelated conditions. Examples include sepsis, lung contusion and drug overdose. The increase in lung water in ARDS occurs as a result of an increase in alveolar capillary permeability and is not due to an increase in hydrostatic forces.

Clinically and radiographically, ARDS closely resembles severe haemodynamic pulmonary oedema due to heart failure. The distinction between these disorders is often apparent from the clinical circumstances associated with the onset of respiratory distress, whereas differentiation by radiographic means alone is often extremely difficult. As in cardiac pulmonary oedema, the increase in lung water associated with ARDS produces interstitial oedema and alveolar collapse, and so the affected lung becomes stiff and the alveolar–arterial oxygen tension difference widens. The central venous pressure and ejection fraction may alter but would not reflect the underlying pathophysiological mechanism. A Swan–Ganz catheter should be placed if the mechanism of oedema formation cannot be discerned with confidence. A pulmonary capillary wedge pressure of less than 18 mmHg favours acute lung injury over haemodynamic pulmonary oedema. In clinical practice, determination of the pulmonary artery wedge pressure is the most helpful investigation for discriminating between ARDS and cardiac failure.

2.9   B: The click and murmur occur earlier in systole when the patient stands up

The systolic click-murmur syndrome is associated with mitral valve prolapse. It occurs in approximately 4% of the normal asymptomatic population. It can place excessive stress on the papillary muscles and lead to ischaemia and chest pain. Although often associated with inferior T-wave changes, the systolic click-murmur syndrome only occasionally results in an ischaemic response to exercise. On standing or during the Valsalva manoeuvre, as the ventricular volume gets smaller, the click and murmur move earlier in systole. Echocardiography reveals mid-systolic prolapse of the posterior mitral leaflet or, occasionally, both mitral leaflets into the left atrium. Asymmetrical hypertrophy of the interventricular septum is a feature of hypertrophic obstructive cardiomyopathy (HOCM). Infective endocarditis prophylaxis is necessary for those patients with a murmur; an isolated mid-systolic click does not merit this.

2.10   A: Bicuspid aortic valve disease

Approximately 1% of the general population has a bicuspid aortic valve defect. The bicuspid aortic valve may function normally throughout life, with late stenosis resulting from fibrocalcific thickening. Aortic stenosis caused by bicuspid valve disease occurs as a result of the increasing calcification and increasing rigidity of the abnormal aortic valve. It is the commonest cause of aortic stenosis. In the congenital form of bicuspid aortic valve disease the cusps are conjoined anteriorly.

2.11   A: Ischaemic heart disease

Mitral stenosis, tricuspid stenosis and secondary pulmonary hypertension due to pulmonary embolism are often associated with right ventricular strain and hypertrophy with partial or complete right bundle branch block. Pericarditis is not associated with bundle branch block.

2.12   E: Barium enema would be advised to exclude colonic malignancy

This patient has *Streptococcus bovis* subacute bacterial endocarditis. *S. bovis* is a Gram-positive coccus. The most common manifestations of *S. bovis* infection are bacteraemia and infective endocarditis.The organism is usually susceptible to penicillin and infection generally responds to the same treatment regimens prescribed for infections due to *S. viridans* – benzylpenicillin, 12–18 million units/24 hours intravenously, given continuously or in divided doses for 4 weeks.

In view of the association between *S. bovis* bacteraemia or infective endocarditis with colonic neoplasia, it is strongly recommended that all adult patients with *S. bovis* bacteraemia undergo an aggressive diagnostic evaluation to search for colonic malignancy. The organism is not generally considered to be part of the normal oral flora although bacteria described as *S. bovis* have been identified in cultures of gingiva or throat in small numbers of individuals. Identification of vegetations on an echocardiogram is diagnostic of subacute bacterial endocarditis.

2.13   B: A 10-mmHg drop in diastolic blood pressure towards the end of pregnancy

Despite an expansion of the plasma volume and cardiac output of 50%, the mean and diastolic blood pressures fall by approximately 15% in pregnancy, owing to a reduction in peripheral vascular resistance. Tachycardia rather than bradycardia is a recognised physiological change during pregnancy. It is a consequence of reduced peripheral vascular resistance and a fall in blood pressure levels. The heart may be slightly enlarged and may be displaced outwards because of the high diaphragm. A pulmonary systolic murmur arising from the high blood flow is common and there may be a physiological third heart sound. Diastolic murmurs are generally pathological and over the mitral area may signify mitral stenosis. The presence of pulsus alternans usually signifies advanced heart failure.

2.14   B: Radiation to the lower jaw

Retrosternal chest pain, though characteristic of ischaemic heart disease, is also encountered in other conditions, such as oesophageal spasm and tracheitis. T-wave inversion in lead III is non-specific and in isolation carries no significance. The ingestion of a heavy meal could precipitate an attack of angina, but could also induce chest pain by causing oesophageal spasm or reflux oesophagitis. Male gender is an independent risk factor for angina and ischaemic heart disease but women also suffer from ischaemic heart disease and alternative causes of retrosternal chest pain manifest in male patients. Chest pain due to angina commonly radiates to the left shoulder and left arm but this does not occur exclusively in angina. In contrast, radiation to the lower jaw (mandible or lower teeth) is the most specific characteristic of anginal pain. Pain above the mandible or below the umbilicus is due to causes other than ischaemic heart disease or angina.

2.15   E: It has a high negative predictive value, so a negative result almost completely excludes venous thromboembolism

D-dimer is a plasmin-mediated fibrin breakdown product and elevated levels in the plasma imply that fibrin has formed and subsequently undergone proteolysis. Several studies have shown that plasma D-dimer levels are elevated in a variety of clotting disorders, including deep venous thrombosis and pulmonary embolism. However, non-thrombotic disorders such as inflammatory disease and postoperative surgical haemostasis can also lead to elevated D-dimer levels. Therefore, D-dimer assays are sensitive for deep venous thrombosis and pulmonary embolism but relatively non-specific – in other words, the presence of normal D-dimer levels helps to exclude these diseases (high negative predictive value) but the presence of elevated levels is non-diagnostic (low positive predictive value). Elevated D-dimer levels are often detected in plasma regardless of the size or the type of blood vessel involved. A ruptured Baker's cyst is associated with an intense inflammatory reaction in the calf, which may lead to activation of the coagulation cascade and even to secondary venous thrombosis.

2.16 D: Brugada syndrome

A family history of cardiac arrest and sudden death, especially at a young age, may suggest a congenital (familial) cardiac disorder. These ECG findings are suggestive of Brugada syndrome. ST-segment elevation in Brugada syndrome is limited to the right precordial leads, slowly down-sloping and followed by negative T waves. It is often associated with conduction delay in the right ventricle, so leading to varying degrees of right bundle branch block.

Brugada syndrome was first described by the Brugada brothers as a distinct clinical entity associated with a high risk of sudden cardiac death (SCD) in 1992. This familial syndrome displays an autosomal dominant mode of inheritance with incomplete penetrance. Missense mutations in the *SCN5A* gene are responsible for significant effects on the cardiac sodium-channel characteristics. Brugada syndrome has a male predominance (8:1) and arrhythmic events tend to manifest before the age of 40. Clinical presentation can vary from syncope to SCD. In some cases, SCD may be the first manifestation of the disease. Self-terminating rapid polymorphic ventricular tachycardias are responsible for repeated episodes of syncope. Clinical reports appear to suggest that SCD occurs commonly during sleep and in the early hours of the morning. An implantable cardioverter defibrillator is the only established effective treatment for the disease in symptomatic patients.

Romano–Ward syndrome is recognised as familial long-QT syndrome, an inherited disorder of myocardial repolarisation in which affected individuals have prolongation of the corrected QT interval on the ECG and a tendency to develop ventricular arrhythmia, leading to syncope, convulsion or sudden death. Wolff–Parkinson–White syndrome is a very rare non-familial cause of sudden cardiac death: a short PR interval and a δ wave are the characteristic ECG changes. ST-segment elevation in leads V1–V3 may be found during acute anterior myocardial infarction. Familial hypercholesterolaemia may explain a similar ischaemic attack in a close relative. In such instances, history and ECG changes of angina pectoris and raised cardiac enzymes are common findings and the differential diagnosis is easily established. A normal echocardiogram virtually excludes the diagnosis of hypertrophic cardiomyopathy.

2.17   A: Atheroembolic disease

Although each of the mentioned options is a valid possible underlying cause behind this presentation, it is clear that the picture is more typical of atheroembolic disease. It is due to cholesterol emboli lodged in peripheral arteries, commonly as a result of angiographic or other surgical vascular procedures. Clearly, the clinical features will depend on the site of embolisation. The most common clinical findings are cutaneous features, renal failure and worsening hypertension. The presence of foot pulses with gangrenous toes should suggest cholesterol embolisation. The retina provides a unique opportunity to visualise the cholesterol emboli. Renal failure may manifest as gradual deterioration of renal function following angiography or may be acute (and may mimic acute dissection of the renal artery during renal angiography). Eosinophilia, eosinophiluria, a raised ESR and hypocomplementaemia have been found in atheroembolic disease.

2.18   A: Constrictive pericarditis

An inspiratory increase in venous pressure (Kussmaul's sign) and a steep *y* descent in the jugular pulse are features of constrictive pericarditis. Pericardial knock in early diastole is often seen in constrictive pericarditis and is not a feature of cardiac tamponade. Both conditions cause failure of either side of the heart and the diastolic pressures in all the cardiac chambers are equalised. A paradoxical pulse and prominent *x* descent in the jugular pulse are more common in tamponade than in constrictive pericarditis.

2.19   D: Right ventricular acute myocardial infarction

Suspect a right ventricular acute myocardial infarction in all patients who present with an inferior wall acute myocardial infarction. Look for the classic triad of distended neck veins, clear lungs and hypotension. These signs emerge as the right heart loses its ability to handle systemic venous return. Right atrial pressure rises and jugular vein distension occurs without pulmonary congestion. When the compromised right ventricle is unable to eject its contents, cardiac output drops, leaving the left ventricle in a state of relative hypovolaemia. Treatment is by rapid loading of intravenous fluid in an attempt to increase the venous return and improve the preload volume, forcing more volume into the left ventricle, which will produce cardiac output that will maintain higher blood pressure and restore tissue perfusion.

Perforated peptic ulcer often presents with epigastric pain and vomiting and might lead to septic shock secondary to an acute abdomen. This manifests with hypotension, tachycardia and reduced urine output; the JVP is not raised and one would not expect to see acute cardiac ischaemic changes on a 12-lead ECG. Raised JVP, hypotension and tachycardia are features of cardiac tamponade; low voltage and electrical alternance are the characteristic ECG abnormalities. Acute aortic regurgitation and acute ventricular septal defect secondary to acute myocardial infarction are often associated with acute pulmonary oedema and a myriad of cardiac and pulmonary physical signs.

2.20   D: Warfarin therapy should be initiated to keep the INR between 2 and 3

Her age and the fact that she is hypertensive put her at increased risk for thromboembolism. Anticoagulant therapy is indicated. Atrial fibrillation is a marker of risk for atherosclerosis and stroke. The current guidelines recommend a ventricular rate of 60–80 bpm at rest during atrial fibrillation as appropriate rate control. Therefore, any medication aimed at rate control, such as digoxin, would not add further to the cardiac performance nor improve any symptoms when she has none. Furthermore, medication aimed at rate conversion and maintenance of sinus rhythm (flecainide, amiodarone) will not improve survival in this group of patients.

Chapter 3

CLINICAL PHARMACOLOGY AND TOXICOLOGY

Answers

3.1   D: Intravenous thiamine

In cases of accidental hypothermia, thiamine may be given empirically to all patients because a patient's history of alcohol abuse may not be available and thiamine has minimal adverse effects. If bedside glucose testing is unavailable, a trial of glucose is warranted because most patients have depleted their glycogen stores, and hypothermia masks the clinical signs of hypoglycaemia. Intravenous antibiotics can be initiated empirically in high-risk groups (neonates, elderly, immunocompromised) because there may be a suboptimal response in the white cell count (WCC) and the C-reactive protein (CRP) despite the presence of overwhelming infection.

Steroid supplementation should not be given empirically to all patients. Stress-dose steroids should be restricted to patients with a history of known adrenal insufficiency and those whose body temperature fails to normalise despite the use of appropriate warming techniques. Most dysrhythmias will correct with warming alone, including the slow atrial fibrillation seen in this patient. A pacemaker is not therefore generally indicated unless a symptomatic slow rhythm persists despite the patient having been warmed, with a core temperature above 35 °C. On the other hand, ventricular fibrillation should be treated with defibrillation and this might need to be repeated. Nasogastric tube insertion should be avoided in all hypothermic patients because of the risk of inducing ventricular fibrillation.

3.2 B: Copper

D-penicillamine is used to reduce the body's copper burden in Wilson's disease.

3.3 A: The baseline CO may exceed 15% in smokers, compared with 1–3% in non-smokers

Carbon monoxide (CO) is one of the most important causes of death from poisoning in many developed countries. The two most common sources of the gas in acute poisonings are motor vehicle exhaust fumes and fumes from domestic gas heaters. The affinity of haemoglobin for CO is 200–250 times greater than its affinity for oxygen. A low baseline level of CO is detectable in everyone. Tobacco smoke is an important source of CO. Blood CO commonly reaches a level of 10% in smokers and may even exceed 15%, compared with 1–3% in non-smokers. CO poisoning in pregnancy has an especially deleterious effect on the fetus, because of the greater sensitivity of the fetus to the harmful effects of the gas. The concentration of carboxyhaemoglobin increases slowly in the fetus and reaches a peak that is 10–15% higher than that in the mother. The exaggerated leftward shift of CO makes tissue hypoxia more severe by causing less oxygen to be released to fetal tissues. Venous blood samples are adequate, although an arterial sample allows for additional determination of coexisting acidosis. CT imaging of the head is not helpful in establishing the diagnosis of CO intoxication and is usually within normal limits. However, it may be used to rule out other conditions that might result in changes in mental status or loss of consciousness.

3.4 C: The plasma paracetamol concentration should be measured urgently

Naloxone is a specific opioid antagonist. It is the only antagonist which reverses the effects of pentazocine overdosage but even at very large doses it is unlikely to counteract the effects of buprenorphine. Administration of naloxone to poisoned opioid addicts may precipitate an acute withdrawal syndrome comprising abdominal cramps, nausea, diarrhoea, piloerection and vasoconstriction. While this is distressing, it is short-lived and seldom severe. In such cases it is advisable to titrate the amount of naloxone given so that life-threatening toxicity is reversed without precipitating significant withdrawal symptoms.

Naloxone may occasionally reverse the CNS toxicity of ethanol and diazepam. In patients who are not obviously addicts, an unexpected response raises the possibility of poisoning with a paracetamol/opioid formulation. The plasma paracetamol concentration should be measured urgently. Patients who have become unconscious as a result of taking an overdose of such combined preparations have also taken sufficient paracetamol to be at risk of severe, but preventable, liver necrosis.

While intravenous administration is the optimum route, there are occasions when venous access is not possible. In such situations naloxone may be instilled down an endotracheal tube or given intramuscularly. Sublingual injection has also been used in shocked patients.

3.5   C: Gentamicin

Aminoglycosides, quinoline antimicrobial drugs, aztreonam and ceftazidime are least active against anaerobic bacteria. These drugs are included in antimicrobial regimes for treating mixed infections, though their role is clearly to suppress the facultative Gram-negative organisms.

The following drugs all have anti-anaerobic activity:

- penicillin
- cephalosporins
- erythromycin
- clindamycin
- tetracycline
- chloramphenicol
- metronidazole.

3.6   A: It reduces protein C levels in the blood

Warfarin competitively inhibits carboxylation of vitamin K-dependent factors. Vitamin K-dependent factors include factors II, VII, IX and X (reverse the year 1972) and protein C. The half-life of warfarin is approximately 44 hours. The level of warfarin in breast milk is too low to be of any clinical significance. Autoimmune thrombocytopenia and osteoporosis are side-effects associated with heparin rather than warfarin.

3.7   B: It has no significant effect on Gram-negative cocci

Vancomycin is bactericidal against several species of Gram-positive cocci but it is less effective against Gram-negative cocci. It acts on multiplying organisms by inhibiting formation of the peptidoglycan component of the cell wall. Vancomycin is poorly absorbed from the gut and it is eliminated by the kidney. Its main side-effect is damage to the auditory portion of the VIIIth cranial nerve.

3.8   E: Acetazolamide

Acetazolamide (a carbonic anhydrase inhibitor) inhibits proximal tubule bicarbonate resorption in a similar fashion to type 2 renal tubular acidosis (RTA). Amiloride acts by inhibiting the sodium channel in the collecting duct, which inhibits renal acid secretion or bicarbonate resorption. All diuretics that promote sodium chloride loss and cause volume depletion are more likely to produce a picture of metabolic alkalosis.

3.9   B: It stimulates the pancreas to release stored insulin

Unlike biguanides, sulphonylureas act primarily by stimulating the β islet cells of the pancreas to release stored insulin. The main mode of action of biguanides is to reduce the absorption of carbohydrate from the gut and to increase the utilisation of glucose in peripheral tissues, as long as insulin is present; these drugs also reduce hepatic gluconeogenesis. Sulphonylurea use is associated with hypoglycaemia, which is sometimes prolonged and may be life-threatening. Biguanides, on the other hand, do not cause clinical hypoglycaemia in normal subjects or in diabetics, but do cause lactic acidosis.

3.10   C: SSRIs have a less profound antimuscarinic effect

Selective serotonin-reuptake inhibitors (SSRIs) are a group of antidepressants that differ from tricyclic antidepressants in that they are less sedative, with weak antimuscarinic effects and low cardiotoxicity. They do not cause weight gain, and the gastrointestinal side-effects, namely diarrhoea, nausea and vomiting, are dose-related. As with tricyclic antidepressants, caution is necessary in prescribing these for epileptic patients. In patients taking MAOIs, a 2-week drug-free period is necessary before commencing treatment with SSRIs.

3.11   C: It is not associated with an increased incidence of late leukaemia

Radioactive iodine is administered as an oral solution or as a capsule of sodium ^{131}I, which is rapidly concentrated in thyroid tissue. The β emissions result in ablation of the gland in 6–18 weeks. The parathyroid gland is not affected because the radiation penetrates only 0.5 mm of tissue. Only 10–15% of patients fail to respond to the first radioiodine treatment and require a second or subsequent dose. Many large studies, including a prospective study of 36,000 patients, have not found an increased risk of cancer or of leukaemia. It is generally accepted that there is an increased risk of exacerbation of Graves' ophthalmopathy during radioactive iodine therapy.

3.12   B: Halothane hepatitis usually becomes evident approximately 7–10 days after anaesthesia

Isoniazid typically induces liver damage in rapid acetylators. With repeated exposure to halothane anaesthesia, the intervals between exposure and clinical manifestations decrease. The mechanism of injury is not known, but an immune mechanism has been postulated. All erythromycins cause a cholestatic reaction in the liver, except for erythromycin stearate. Chlorpromazine and flucloxacillin also induce a cholestatic reaction, while allopurinol, phenytoin and hydralazine usually cause liver granulomas.

3.13   E: Dipyridamole

Dipyridamole is a weak antiplatelet agent that acts by increasing the cellular concentration of cAMP. It inhibits the phosphodiesterase enzyme which converts cAMP to inactive 5'AMP. Elevated levels of cAMP and cGMP inhibit activation and aggregation of platelets. Aspirin is a potent inhibitor of platelet cyclooxygenase. This is an enzyme that converts arachidonic acid to thromboxane A_2 (TXA_2), a strong platelet agonist. Because the platelet has no protein synthetic apparatus the effects of aspirin are irreversible and last for the life of the platelet (8–10 days). The antiplatelet effect of clopidogrel, like ticlopidine, results from antagonism of a platelet ADP receptor, P2T, resulting in inhibition of platelet activation. This antagonism is non-competitive, irreversible, and results in 50–70% inhibition of fibrinogen binding.

Regardless of the mechanism of activation, the final common pathway for platelet aggregation is the cross-linking of platelets through fibrinogen. Abciximab is a humanised monoclonal antibody. It is a selective glycoprotein IIb/IIIa receptor antagonist.

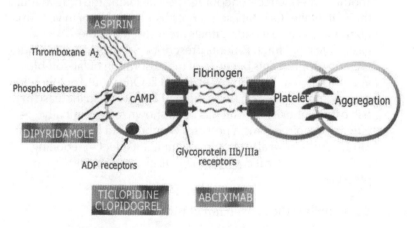

Platelet aggregation factors and antiplatelet sites of action.

3.14 D: They decrease the heart rate and myocardial contractility

The cardiovascular effects of β-adrenoceptor blockade depend on the amount of sympathetic tone present. The chief cardiac effects result from reduction of the sympathetic drive – reduced heart rate (automaticity) and reduced myocardial contractility (rate of rise of pressure in the ventricle). This will lead to reduced cardiac output and an overall fall in oxygen consumption. Beta-blockers cause a rise in peripheral vascular resistance due to the unopposed α-adrenoceptor effects (vasoconstriction). This last effect has no role in alleviating angina.

3.15 A: It prevents fat absorption from the intestine

Orlistat (Xenical®) therapy effectively promotes weight loss and improves comorbidities in obese patients. Orlistat operates by preventing the absorption of fat molecules in the intestinal tract. Approximately 30% of fat that would otherwise have been absorbed passes straight through the bowel and is excreted in the faeces. As a result, it can cause 'fatty stools', urgency and increased frequency of defecation, often with anal leakage or oily spotting. These effects encourage people taking the drug to limit their fat intake. Orlistat itself is not absorbed, except in very small quantities, and so its side-effects are restricted to the gastrointestinal tract. Patients prescribed orlistat may also require vitamin supplements because of malabsorption of fat-soluble vitamins such as vitamins A, D, K and E. One would not therefore expect improvement in bone mineral density or an increase in the risk of thrombosis. Orlistat has been shown to be clinically efficacious in reducing a person's weight over a period of a year. Study results have also shown a significant effect in reducing fasting glucose, total cholesterol, LDL cholesterol and blood pressure.

3.16 E: It inhibits the conversion of T4 to T3

Propylthiouracil (PTU) and carbimazole are derivatives of thiourea. Both inhibit the organification of iodine in the thyroid gland as their major mechanism of action. Neither drug affects iodine trapping, nor does either inhibit the release of preformed thyroid hormone. PTU, but not carbimazole, is an inhibitor of T4 to T3 conversion, giving it a modest therapeutic advantage over the latter agent. The quantities of PTU in the breast milk of mothers receiving therapeutic doses of PTU are not great enough to cause impairment of an infant's thyroid function. It seems likely that nursing mothers could take PTU at low doses, though the infant could still be at risk of non-thyroid complications of this drug. Significant amounts of carbimazole are secreted in milk, so it should not be given to nursing mothers. Thiourea derivatives have several side-effects, including a maculopapular rash, hepatocellular damage and vasculitis. The most serious side-effect of both agents is agranulocytosis. Carbimazole is approximately 15 times more potent than PTU.

3.17   A: Doxorubicin

Anthracyclines (doxorubicin) are particularly known for causing cumulative, dose-dependent cardiotoxicity which manifests as impaired left ventricular function and congestive cardiac failure. Cyclophosphamide is an alkylating agent which is metabolised to the active form in the liver. Acrolein, a product, may be responsible for the common side-effect of haemorrhagic cystitis. Chronic liver disease is encountered more with methotrexate therapy. *Cis*-platinum (cisplatin) is a heavy metal compound often used to treat testicular and ovarian tumours. It causes nephrotoxicity in 30% of patients, with damage to the distal tubules and collecting ducts leading to persistent magnesium-wasting. The most important side-effect of bleomycin is progressive interstitial pulmonary fibrosis with bibasal pulmonary infiltrates seen on chest X-ray. Vincristine is a vinca alkaloid and when used on a weekly basis there is a risk of progressive peripheral neuropathy. There is greater improvement in the sensory changes than in the motor changes after discontinuation of vincristine.

3.18   E: An insulin sensitiser which decreases peripheral insulin resistance

The thiazolidinediones (TZDs) comprise a major new group of drugs which includes rosiglitazone (Avandia®) and pioglitazone (Actos®). These drugs exert their effect by activating the peroxisome proliferation-activated receptor-γ (PPARγ). This nuclear receptor influences the differentiation of fibroblasts into adipocytes and lowers free fatty acid levels. Clinically, their major effect is to decrease peripheral insulin resistance, although at higher doses they may also decrease hepatic glucose production. Although acting at a different site from metformin, both rosiglitazone and metformin appear to function as insulin sensitisers and require the presence of insulin for their effects. In contrast to metformin, the effects of pioglitazone may be progressive over time, and its full hypoglycaemic potency may not be achieved until the patient has received 12 weeks of therapy. Unlike sulphonylureas and repaglinide (a benzoic acid derivative), TZDs have no stimulatory effect on insulin secretion. Acarbose acts locally in the small intestine by inhibiting α-glucosidase enzymes: this action slows digestion of ingested carbohydrates, delays glucose absorption, and reduces the increase in postprandial blood glucose.

3.19   B: Doxazosin

Prazosin, terazosin, and doxazosin are peripheral postsynaptic α_1-adrenergic blockers that act on veins and arterioles. Losartan blocks angiotensin II receptors and therefore interferes with the renin–angiotensin system, perhaps more completely than the angiotensin-converting enzyme (ACE) inhibitors. Losartan does not block the degradation of bradykinin, which perhaps explains why it does not cause a dry irritating cough. Methyldopa and clonidine reduce sympathetic nervous activity by stimulating the presynaptic α_2-adrenergic receptors in the brainstem. Methyldopa acts primarily on the brainstem vasomotor centre, causing the release of a false neurotransmitter (α-methylnoradrenaline) which enhances the agonist effect on CNS α_2-adrenoceptors that mediates inhibition of the sympathetic outflow. It results in reduction of peripheral vascular resistance with reduction of blood pressure. Its action on the peripheral adrenergic ending is clinically insignificant and so it does not cause postural hypotension. Minoxidil causes direct relaxation of vascular smooth muscle and acts mainly on arterial resistance rather than on venous capacitance vessels, as evidenced by the lack of postural effects. It unfortunately produces significant hypertrichosis and fluid retention and therefore is mainly limited to patients with severe hypertension and renal insufficiency.

3.20   B: Dilatation of systemic veins

Glyceryl trinitrate products are both venous capacitance dilators and coronary and systemic artery dilators and they have complex beneficial effects in patients with coronary artery disease. Administration of glyceryl trinitrate results in dilatation of systemic veins and a decrease in myocardial wall tension and oxygen demand. This is accompanied by dilatation of large and medium-sized coronary arteries with increased coronary blood flow to the subendocardium. Glyceryl trinitrate reduces the afterload and preload and improves coronary perfusion. Due to the peripheral blood pooling, it reduces the ventricular volume and increases ventricular compliance.

3.21   B: Increased bradykinin concentration

The mechanisms responsible for ACE inhibitor-related cough are not fully understood. It affects up to 20% of patients and is commoner in women. It is thought to be due to increased production of bradykinins and/or substance P, which activate the cough reflex. The cough usually begins within 1–2 months after starting therapy. It is dry, persistent, and mostly non-productive, and it is often described as a 'tickling in the throat'. It may occur more frequently when a person reclines, and it usually resolves 5–7 days after the drug is discontinued. Angiotensin II-receptor blockers are distinct from the ACE inhibitors in that they have no effect on angiotensin-converting enzyme. Rather, they block the diverse physiological effects of angiotensin II by specifically blocking angiotensin II tissue receptors. These drugs are not associated with an increase in circulating bradykinins, so theoretically they should cause less of a problem with cough.

3.22   C: It has calcium-channel-blocking properties

Amiodarone has a high iodine content (40% of its weight); it provides the body with approximately 12 times the average daily requirement when given at a dose of 200 mg/day. This means an increased iodine load with possible altered thyroid handling of iodine, with the prospect of hypothyroidism (the Wolff–Chaikoff effect) or hyperthyroidism due to increased conversion of iodine to thyroxine. Amiodarone can directly cause both sinus bradycardia and atrioventricular block, due primarily to its calcium-channel-blocking activity. Of great potential concern is the prolongation of the QT interval due to blockage of the potassium channels. It is used effectively for both ventricular and supraventricular tachyarrhythmias. Corneal microdeposits occur in most patients receiving long-term amiodarone therapy. This complication is dose-dependent and is reversible when the drug is discontinued. The microdeposits are caused by the secretion of amiodarone by the lacrimal gland; they accumulate on the corneal surface. Amiodarone inhibits cytochrome P450 in the liver, thus inhibiting the metabolism of other drugs. This can raise digoxin levels by as much as 100%, and so the digoxin dose should be reduced by 50% when commencing amiodarone. Amiodarone might also displace digoxin from its protein-binding sites, thus increasing its levels in the serum.

3.23   A: It acts by direct inhibition of thrombin

Ximelagatran is an oral direct thrombin inhibitor (DTI) which blocks the formation of fibrin without a quantitative effect on the prothrombin time or partial thromboplastin time. It is not a vitamin K-dependent factor. Studies have demonstrated that ximelagatran is not inferior to warfarin. Moreover, ximelagatran has a more rapid onset of action than warfarin (showing its anticoagulant effect within 1 hour after oral administration). It can be administered twice daily in a fixed-dose regime, without any need for monitoring. There have been no known drug interactions with ximelagatran and it is not metabolised by the hepatic cytochrome P450 system. For these reasons, orally active DTIs such as ximelagatran are likely to become the standard for long-term anticoagulation.

In a small percentage of patients (0.5%) ximelagatran may cause mild elevation of both alanine aminotransferase (ALT) and bilirubin levels and the liver function tests may need to be monitored, especially during the first 6 months of therapy. Bleeding complications occur less frequently than with warfarin therapy. There is no direct antidote for ximelagatran. It is largely eliminated through the kidneys, and so caution should be exercised in individuals with renal impairment.

3.24   C: Sublingual glyceryl trinitrate

Sildenafil citrate (Viagra®) is indicated for the treatment of erectile dysfunction. Large and sudden decreases in systemic blood pressure have been reported in a substantial number of patients taking sildenafil citrate combined with glyceryl trinitrate.

Sildenafil is a selective inhibitor of cGMP-specific phosphodiesterase type 5 (PDE5) enzyme, and its use leads to an increase in the levels of cyclic guanosine monophosphate (cGMP). By inhibiting PDE5, sildenafil enhances the normal physiological action of nitric oxide (NO) and cGMP. The physiological mechanism responsible for erection of the penis involves the release of NO in the corpus cavernosum in response to sexual stimulation. NO activates the enzyme guanylate cyclase, which results in locally increased levels of cGMP, producing smooth muscle relaxation in the corpus cavernosum and leading to an erection adequate for sexual intercourse. However, sildenafil may cause smooth muscle relaxation, not only in the corpus cavernosum, but also in systemic vascular smooth muscle. This is why it should not be used with organic nitrates such as glyceryl trinitrate patches or sublingual tablets – the combination may lower the blood pressure. There have been many reports on sildenafil citrate in which there was a fatal outcome.

3.25   C: 10–30% of the inhaled dose of insulin is absorbed into the circulation

Around 10–30% of the inhaled dose of insulin is absorbed into the circulation, and so approximately 100 times the dose of subcutaneous insulin is required to achieve similar glycaemic control. Cigarette smoking increases absorption of inhaled insulin. A bedtime subcutaneus Ultratard® insulin injection plus preprandial inhaled insulin is required to give similar glucose control to the usual subcutaneous insulin regimens of two to three daily insulin injections. Inhaled insulin peaks at least as rapidly as a fast-acting analogue injected subcutaneously, and has a longer duration of effect. Studies to date have shown no effect on pulmonary function (on spirometry, lung volumes, diffusion capacity or oxygen saturation).

3.26   E: Bioavailability immediately following intravenous injection of a drug

Renal failure disturbs virtually every kinetic parameter, including gastric absorption, hepatic metabolism of some drugs, protein binding and volume of distribution. The bioavailability of an intravenously administered drug is 100% and does not change in renal failure.

3.27   A: The decline of drug concentration in the plasma from the arterial to the venous side of the kidney

The extraction ratio is a measure of how much drug is extracted from the plasma by the kidney. It determines the clearance (= renal plasma flow × extraction ratio). The time during which the concentration of a drug in the plasma halves is the half-life. The proportion of an orally administered drug reaching the circulation is the bioavailability.

3.28   E: Ciclosporin therapy

Bartter's syndrome is associated with hypokalaemia resulting from a number of inherited defects of renal function. Corticosteroids are associated with hypokalaemia due to their mineralocorticoid effects. Liquorice inhibits 11-hydroxysteroid dehydrogenase, causing potassium-wasting from the distal tubule. Liddle's syndrome is a rare condition, comprising hypokalaemia, hypertension and low aldosterone levels. Ciclosporin use can lead to an increase in blood pressure and renal impairment with hyperkalaemia. Some renal transplant patients treated with ciclosporin run serum potassium concentrations in the range 6.0–7.1 mmol/l. This effect is probably a variant of hyporeninaemic hypoaldosteronism and is responsive to fludrocortisone.

3.29 C: Haemodialysis

This patient is apparently suffering from chronic rather than acute lithium toxicity. Chronic use of lithum may cause an increase in the half-life of the drug over time. Patients on chronic therapy are therefore more prone to develop toxicity. Other factors should be considered, such as renal impairment and concomitant use of drugs such as NSAIDs and diuretics. This patient's presentation is an emergency and he should be managed in an Intensive Care Unit. Haemodialysis has been the mainstay of therapy in severe lithium intoxication, although the specific indications are poorly established. In general, consider dialysis in patients with chronic toxicity and serum lithium concentrations higher than 4 mmol/l; also consider dialysis in unstable patients on chronic treatment with lithium levels higher than 2.5 mmol/l.

Features of mild to moderate lithium intoxication include thirst, tremor, polyuria, diarrhoea, vomiting and, in severe cases, impairment of consciousness, hypertonia and convulsions. Toxicity is usually associated with levels >1.5 mmol/l. All patients with lithium poisoning should have their lithium levels, U&Es and plasma osmolality measured.

Methionine is used as an antidote for paracetamol poisoning. Activated charcoal adsorbs drugs in the gut and increases removal of drugs from the body by interfering with enterohepatic and entero-enteric circulation of the drug; it is generally more effective in the acute overdose setting. Forced diuresis could be helpful as lithium is eliminated solely through the kidneys, but in serious and emergency situations, as in this patient, it might not be appropriate to rely on this form of intervention as a sole therapy. Methylprednisolone has no role in the treatment of chronic lithium toxicity (cerebral oedema is not the mechanism responsible for the cerebral manifestations in lithium toxicity).

3.30 C: Allopurinol is a known cause

The kidneys are usually enlarged in acute interstitial nephritis. Drugs are the most important factors in the aetiology of this condition, which is immune-mediated. Haematuria and renal impairment are constant features and should be monitored to assess the patient's response to treatment.

3.31   C: Punctate basophilic stippling on peripheral blood film examination

Lead poisoning can occur through ingestion, inhalation and direct skin contact. Numerous occupations entail potentially significant exposure, eg miners, welders, storage battery workers. Pottery workers are particularly heavily exposed. The exact pathogenesis of lead colic remains uncertain. In part, it appears to be due to the direct effect of lead on intestinal smooth muscle. Lead interferes with a variety of red cell enzymes, leading to red cell abnormalities which include punctate basophilic stippling and 'clover leaf' morphology. The peripheral neuropathy, which is seen in adult patients, is exclusively motor. Interstitial nephritis is the characteristic lesion in the kidneys. A gingival blue-black or grey line is found in up to 20% of adult patients but is an infrequent finding in children.

Chapter 4

DERMATOLOGY

Answers

4.1   B: Erythema gyratum repens

Erythema gyratum repens is associated with malignancy in as many as 80% of patients. Among visceral malignancies, the lung is the most common site. Most patients with erythema gyratum repens develop the eruption before the symptoms of the tumour itself. The time interval between the eruption of erythema gyratum repens and the detection of the tumour can range from simultaneous presentation to up to 6 years after the rash has appeared.

Erythema marginatum is a serpiginous, flat, non-scarring, painless rash. It is transient, sometimes lasting for less than a day. It occurs in less than 5% of patients with rheumatic fever, but is considered a major Jones criterion when it does occur. Erythema chronicum migrans is the rash that is associated with early Lyme disease. It usually occurs 3–32 days after a tick bite. There is a gradual expansion of redness around the site of the tick bite. The advancing border is raised, warm, red or bluish-red and ringlike. The ring appears to grow and can become quite large (up to 24 inches). Erythema multiforme lesions are known as 'target' or 'iris' skin lesions and are less than 3 cm in diameter. The cutaneous lesions are typically symmetrical and involve the extensor surfaces of the extremities. It is often associated with herpes simplex infection or drug reactions to agents such as sulpha drugs or penicillin. Erythema nodosum is characterised by tender, red bumps, usually found on the shins. It is commonly associated with streptococcal infections, sarcoidosis and leprosy.

4.2   C: Chronic myeloid leukaemia

Pyoderma gangrenosum is characterised by deep, red, necrotic ulcers with undermined, violaceous, oedematous borders. These lesions typically evolve over the lower limbs and are encountered in the following conditions:

- inflammatory bowel disease (ulcerative colitis, Crohn's disease)
- rheumatoid arthritis, Wegener's granulomatosis
- lymphoma
- myeloproliferative disorders, eg myelogenous and myeloblastic leukaemia, myeloma, myeloid metaplasia, polycythaemia rubra vera, monoclonal gammopathy.

Tuberculosis is associated with lupus vulgaris and erythema induratum. Leprosy is associated with erythema leprosum. Cushing's syndrome is associated with skin stria and easy bruising. These conditions are not associated with pyoderma gangrenosum. Sulphonamide therapy is associated with various skin eruptions, including erythema nodosum, but again is not associated with pyoderma gangrenosum.

4.3   D: Addison's disease

Vitiligo is a circumscribed hypomelanosis of progressively enlarging melanotic macules in an asymmetric distribution around body orifices and over bony prominences. It is familial in 90% of cases. White hairs are common in the vitiliginous areas. Most patients with vitiligo are healthy, although there is an association with certain autoimmune diseases, such as alopecia areata, Addison's disease, thyroid diseases, pernicious anaemia and diabetes mellitus. Nelson's disease, amiodarone therapy and chronic renal failure are associated with hyperpigmentation. Hyperparathyroidism is not associated with a specific skin lesion.

4.4   A: Herpes simplex infection

Stevens–Johnson syndrome is an immunological reaction in the skin and mucous membranes characterised by iris skin lesions (erythema multiforme) and extensive bulla formation in the mouth and conjunctivae. The commonest disease association is with a preceding herpes simplex or *Mycoplasma pneumoniae* infection. Other causes include drug sensitivity (sulphonamides, penicillins, barbiturates, phenytoin and possibly the contraceptive pill).

4.5   E: Porphyria cutanea tarda

Photo-related conditions occur in the typical distribution of light-exposed areas, which should make the diagnosis apparent. Maximum changes therefore occur over the forehead, malar eminences, bridge of the nose and pinna of the ears, with sparing of the upper lip (shaded by the nose), periorbital areas and submental region. The 'V' of the neck, dorsum of the hands and forearms are often involved, with a sharp demarcation where clothing and watchbands cover the skin.

Causes include:

*   drugs, eg sulphonamides, phenothiazines, thiazides, amiodarone, quinidine, quinine
*   immune disorders, eg lupus (systemic and discoid)
*   metabolic conditions, eg porphyria cutanea tarda, erythropoietic protoporphyria and pellagra (nicotinic acid deficiency) – but not acute intermittent porphyria.

4.6   D: Psoriasis

The Koebner phenomenon occurs in certain skin diseases that tend to evolve new skin lesions after traumatic injuries in areas of apparently normal skin. Lichen planus, pemphigus vulgaris, molluscum contagiosum and vitiligo are associated with this phenomenon. Other causes include psoriasis and warts. Herpes simplex and other skin infections are not associated with this phenomenon.

4.7   E: Granuloma inguinale

Calymmatobacterium granulomatis is a Gram-negative bacillus that reproduces within neutrophils, plasma cells and histiocytes, causing the infected white cells to rupture, with the release of 20–30 organisms. The key features are a primary, painless indurated nodule that progresses to a heaped-up ulcer, and the presence of infected mononuclear cells containing many

Donovan bodies. The infection is endemic in Australia, India, the Caribbean and Africa, and transmission is associated with unprotected sexual intercourse. Treatment is with tetracycline or ampicillin, and patients are advised to refrain from sexual intercourse until the lesion has healed. Relapse is common and routine annual or 6-monthly follow-up is advised.

4.8   C: Dermatitis herpetiformis

Dermatitis herpetiformis presents with this clinical picture, commonly in early adulthood. HLA associations (B8, DR3, DQ2 in 80–90% of cases) are similar to those for coeliac disease. Skin biopsy reveals subepidermal blisters with neutrophil microabscesses in the dermal papillae. There is positive staining for IgA in the dermal papillae and patchy granular IgA along the basement membrane. In this case, where there is a history of diarrhoea, there is likely to be villous atrophy on jejunal biopsy. Treatment is with a gluten-free diet and control of the skin manifestations may be achieved with either dapsone or sulphonamides. Dapsone may rarely be associated with liver pathology, polyneuropathy and aplastic anaemia, so regular monitoring of both liver biochemistry and the blood count is necessary.

4.9   A: Alopecia areata

Alopecia areata is defined as a loss of hair that leaves single or multiple, discrete, often round, areas of shiny baldness on the scalp (most common), in the beard area, or in any hair-bearing part of the body. A sign of disease activity is the presence of broken hairs at the advancing edge of the lesion that look like exclamation marks. These are very short hairs that taper and become depigmented nearer the scalp – they are in the telogen (resting) phase. Nail dystrophy should always be looked for, which takes the form of very fine pitting and is much finer than psoriatic nail pitting. Alopecia areata is considered to be an autoimmune disease, mainly due to its association with other autoimmune diseases, such as vitiligo, thyroid disease, pernicious anaemia, rheumatoid arthritis and diabetes, but no specific antibody has yet been identified. Approximately a third of patients have a positive family history, implying that a genetic component is involved. Many patients experience hair regrowth within 9–12 months. Treating any associated underlying autoimmune disease does not appear to have any positive effect on the alopecia. Steroids, minoxidil, PUVA (psoralen-ultraviolet A) and contact allergen therapy may be useful. No scarring occurs with this form of hair loss

Other causes of hair loss associated with scarring include discoid lupus erythematosus, lichen planus, scleroderma and radiodermatitis, in which the hair follicle is destroyed and signs of inflammation are present. The scalp is atrophic with absent hair follicles in the patches of hair loss and regrowth never occurs. Discoid lupus erythematosus lesions comprise well-defined plaques of erythema with scaling, atrophy and follicular plugging, which affect light-exposed areas of the body and are exacerbated by sunlight. Trichotillomania is the self-inflicted pulling out of one's hair. It is differentiated from alopecia areata by the patterns of irregular hair loss and the fact that growing hairs are always present: hairs cannot be extracted until they are long enough to be seen or caught hold of. Patches of hair loss tend to be unilateral and on the same side as the dominant hand. Telogen effluvium is a transitory (2–4 months), generalised, diffuse hair loss over the scalp with an increased number of hairs in the resting phase of the growth cycle. It is associated with high fever, stress, malnutrition, surgery and oral contraceptives, or may follow childbirth. Scaling and broken hairs are found in patients with fungal infections (tinea capitis) and fungal spores or hyphae are visible on microscopic examination of hair specimens.

4.10   D: Pregnancy should be avoided during and for 1 month after treatment

Isotretinoin is indicated for the treatment of severe inflammatory acne. However, it causes marked dryness of the skin and mucous membranes, especially the lips, and can result in minor nosebleeds. Because of its potential teratogenic effects, pregnancy must be excluded prior to its initiation and during treatment, as well as for 1 month after treatment has finished. Other side-effects are paronychia, meatitis in men and contact lens problems due to dryness of the eyes. Abnormalities of serum lipids and liver function tests should be excluded before treatment and these should also be checked after 4 weeks (and perhaps again after 8 weeks) of treatment.

Chapter 5

ENDOCRINOLOGY AND METABOLIC DISORDERS

Answers

5.1 D: Medullary-cell carcinoma

Medullary-cell carcinoma can be associated with
hyperparathyroidism as part of the multiple endocrine neoplasia
(MEN) syndrome. The other conditions mentioned are associated
with idiopathic hypoparathyroidism, which may be associated
with other autoimmune diseases. This type of hypoparathyroidism
is called 'multiple endocrine deficiency autoimmune candidiasis'
(MEDAC). Mucocutanous candidiasis and Addison's disease are
commonly associated with this disorder. DiGeorge syndrome is
characterised by the absence of the parathyroid gland and tetany
in neonates. Functional hypoparathyroidism occurs in patients
with severe and prolonged hypomagnesaemia of whatever cause.
Magnesium is required for the release of PTH; it also promotes
PTH actions on target tissues.

5.2 E: Bartter's syndrome

Bartter's syndrome is associated with hypokalaemia. Hypertension
is not a feature of this disorder.

Hypertension in association with hypokalaemia is encountered in
the following conditions:

- renovascular disease
- renin-secreting tumours
- mineralocorticoid and glucocorticoid excess, Cushing's

syndrome, Conn's syndrome, congenital adrenal hyperplasia, chronic liquorice ingestion and other adrenal adenomas and carcinomas
* Liddle's syndrome, a rare autosomal dominant disorder of sodium channels in the collecting tubules with a primary increase in sodium resorption and, in most cases, potassium loss.

5.3   C: Conn's syndrome

Mineralocorticoid excess causes metabolic alkalosis in Conn's syndrome. Spironolactone therapy is used to treat Conn's syndrome. Thiazides, loop diuretics and vomiting all cause a metabolic alkalosis through reduction of the extracellular volume and hypokalaemia.

Addison's disease is usually associated with hyperkalaemia and mild metabolic acidosis. However, if persistent vomiting is a feature, mild metabolic alkalosis may occur. Acetazolamide therapy and chronic diarrhoea are associated with a mild metabolic acidosis.

5.4   C: Myxoedema

Galactorrhoea is the non-puerperal expression of milk. Hyperprolactinaemia causes galactorrhoea and amenorrhoea, and may result from a prolactin-secreting pituitary tumour or hyperplasia. In acromegaly, a third of patients have mild elevation of prolactin levels resulting in galactorrhoea, amenorrhoea and decreased libido. A similar elevation of prolactin levels occurs in a small percentage of patients with primary hypothyroidism. Sheehan's syndrome is a primary hypopituitarism due to ischaemic necrosis of the pituitary gland caused by postpartum haemorrhage; it is characterised by failure of postpartum lactation and failure to resume normal cyclic menstruation. Turner's syndrome (ovarian dysgenesis) causes primary amenorrhoea with poor development of the breast. Bromocriptine is a dopaminergic agent that has an inhibitory effect on prolactin and is frequently used to treat hyperprolactinaemia.

5.5   D: Pretibial myxoedema

Exophthalmos and pretibial myxoedema are features of Graves' disease. Proximal muscle weakness and myasthenia gravis (like other autoimmune diseases) are recognised associations of thyrotoxicosis but peripheral neuropathy is not a well-recognised feature. Hair loss, weight gain and menorrhagia are features of hypothyroidism.

5.6   A: 24-hour urine catecholamines

A current or past medical history of medullary thyroid carcinoma should always raise the suspicion of a possible familial neoplasia syndrome. This disorder is known to be linked to the multiple endocrine neoplasia (MEN) group of disorders. When medullary thyroid carcinoma and hyperparathyroidism manifest in the same patient a possible diagnosis of MEN 2A should be considered. MEN 2A is an autosomal dominant disorder which comprises medullary thyroid carcinoma and variable prevalences of hyperparathyroidism and phaeochromocytoma. Tests to investigate for phaeochromocytoma are therefore the most appropriate next step in this patient. MEN 2A phaeochromocytoma must be detected prior to any operation: the phaeochromocytoma should be removed first to remove the risk of severe hypertensive episodes while the thyroid or parathyroid is being operated on. Patients with MEN 2B are affected by medullary thyroid carcinoma, phaeochromocytoma and other features, but do not have parathyroid involvement.

A high gastrin level is a marker of pancreatic gastrinoma and a raised prolactin is a feature of pituitary prolactinoma. Both conditions are features of MEN 1 (parathyroid adenoma, pituitary and pancreatic tumours) and not MEN 2A. A serum angiotensin-converting enzyme level would be helpful to confirm sarcoidosis as the cause of hypercalcaemia. Similarly, serum protein electrophoresis would confirm the diagnosis of multiple myeloma. However, the parathyroid hormone level is usually suppressed in hypercalcaemia associated with both these disorders.

5.7   C: Surgery can be performed safely in the second trimester

Transplacental passage of stimulating thyroid-stimulating hormone-receptor autoantibodies causes fetal and neonatal hyperthyroidism, even long after maternal thyrotoxicosis has resolved clinically. Carbimazole and propylthiouracil form the mainstay of drug treatment; both cross the placenta and doses should therefore be minimised to avoid fetal hypothyroidism and goitre. Surgery may be performed safely in the second trimester, but is usually reserved for treating pressure symptoms secondary to goitre or in cases of failed medical treatment. Although antithyroid drugs may enter breast milk, breastfeeding is permissible when low doses are used.

5.8   D: Aspirin overdose

This patient's deep-sighing respiration and low bicarbonate level are indicative of underlying metabolic acidosis. There are two types of metabolic acidosis, depending on the anion gap values: high anion gap metabolic acidosis or normal anion gap metabolic acidosis. One way to calculate the anion gap is to add the number of chloride and bicarbonate anions and subtract them from the number of sodium and potassium cations:

$$([Na^+] + [K^+]) - ([HCO_3^-] + [Cl^-]) = \text{anion gap}$$

The normal level of anion gap is generally considered to be between 12 mmol/l and 16 mmol/l. An anion gap exceeding 24 mmol/l suggests the presence of metabolic acidosis.

Causes of a high anion gap metabolic acidosis include:

* ketoacidosis
* renal failure
* intoxication, eg with ethylene glycol, methanol, paraldehyde, salicylates.

Causes of a normal anion gap metabolic acidosis include:

* gastrointestinal alkali loss, eg through diarrhoea, ileostomy, colostomy
* renal tubular acidosis types 1, 2 and 4
* interstitial renal disease
* ureterosigmoidostomy
* acetazolamide
* ingestion of ammonium chloride.

This patient's anion gap is 30.5 mmol/l and he has a high anion gap metabolic acidosis. The only possible explanation for his metabolic abnormality is aspirin overdose. Persistent vomiting is associated with metabolic alkalosis. Hyperventilation is often associated with respiratory alkalosis.

5.9   B: 50% will go on to develop maturity-onset diabetes mellitus

Gestational diabetes is defined as diabetes mellitus diagnosed for the first time during pregnancy, which remits after pregnancy. It tends to recur in a subsequent pregnancy in 40% of cases. Approximately 50% will develop maturity-onset diabetes mellitus. There is increased risk of macrosomia and of neonatal hypoglycaemia but there is no increased risk of congenital malformation.

5.10   B: Rhabdomyolysis

Hypophosphataemia leads to depletion of intracellular 2,3-diphosphoglycerate (2,3-DPG) and of ATP. The energy metabolism of the cell may become inadequate to maintain the integrity of its membrane and this may lead to damage or dysfunction of various tissues. Examples of the effects of such damage include:

- red blood cell haemolysis
- white blood cell and platelet dysfunction
- muscle weakness and rhabdomyolysis
- central nervous system dysfunction and peripheral neuropathy
- osteomalacia and rickets.

Hyperphosphataemia, on the other hand, is associated with metastatic calcifications. Carpopedal spasm is a feature associated with low serum calcium levels. Constipation is a feature of hypercalcaemia. Cardiac rhythm abnormalities may be a feature of low potassium and/or magnesium levels.

5.11   B: Apoprotein C-II

Dietary triglycerides in cholesterol are packaged by gastrointestinal epithelial cells into large lipoprotein particles called 'chylomicrons'. After secretion into the intestinal lymph and passage into the general circulation, chylomicrons bind to the enzyme lipoprotein lipase, which is located on endothelial surfaces. This enzyme is activated by a protein contained in the chylomicron, apoprotein C-II, liberating free fatty acids and monoglycerides, which then pass through the endothelial cells and enter adipocyte or muscle cells.

Complete inactivation of either lipoprotein lipase or apoprotein C-II as a result of the inheritance of two defective copies of the relevant gene therefore results in an accumulation of chylomicrons (type I lipoprotein elevation) due to the failure of conversion to the chylomicron remnant particle. Patients with familial lipoprotein lipase deficiency usually present in infancy with recurrent attacks of abdominal pain caused by pancreatitis. They also have eruptive xanthomas resulting from triglyceride deposition. Treatment should consist of a low-fat diet that may be supplemented by medium-chain triglycerides, which are not incorporated into chylomicrons. The absence of functional apoprotein C-II, with consequent failure to activate lipoprotein lipase, presents with a similar phenotype, although the affected patients are typically detected at a somewhat later age than are patients with familial lipoprotein lipase deficiency.

5.12   E: Vitamin D deficiency

The combination of hypocalcaemia and hypophosphataemia points to the diagnosis of osteomalacia and vitamin D deficiency. Dietary deficiency and malabsorption are common causes of vitamin D deficiency. Primary hyperparathyroidism and hypervitaminosis D are associated with hypercalcaemia rather than hypocalcaemia. Paget's disease is associated with increased risk of fracture and increased serum alkaline phosphatase activity, but the serum calcium is usually within normal limits. Osteoporosis is the most common cause of fracture of neck of femur but is not associated with any specific abnormality in the standard bone biochemistry profile.

5.13   B: Renal tubular acidosis

The causes of hypokalaemia include:

1   Inadequate dietary intake.

2   Excessive renal loss:

  • Conn's syndrome

- Bartter's syndrome
- diuretic therapy
- metabolic alkalosis
- gentamicin therapy
- amphotericin therapy
- renal tubular acidosis.

3 Excessive gastrointestinal loss (vomiting and diarrhoea).

Addison's disease, spironolactone therapy, metabolic acidosis and haemolytic anaemia are associated with an increased serum potassium concentration.

5.14 B: Primary hyperparathyroidism

Treatment of severe hypercalcaemia (>3 mmol/l) should be started immediately as the condition is life-threatening. The mainstay of therapy is a regimen of hydration, initially with normal saline, plus forced diuresis using furosemide. Corticosteroids (eg 300 mg of cortisone or 60 mg of prednisolone), given daily, are effective in the treatment of hypercalcaemia of non-parathyroid origin. Treating the primary cause would prevent further recurrence.

5.15 C: Familial dysbetalipoproteinaemia

Palmar xanthomata, which are planar xanthomata in the palmar creases, are virtually pathognomonic of type III hyperlipoproteinaemia, which is also known as 'familial dysbetalipoproteinaemia'.

5.16 A: Acanthosis nigricans

Insulin resistance is defined as a subclinical response to endogenous or exogenous insulin. In the context of diabetes mellitus, it manifests as persistent hyperglycaemia despite high doses of insulin. Features suggestive of insulin resistance include acanthosis nigricans, lipodystrophy, hyperandrogenism (polycystic ovary syndrome), hypertension and ischaemic heart disease. Peripheral neuropathy and the other manifestations listed in the question are recognised complications of diabetes mellitus and are not directly related to insulin resistance.

5.17   E: Necrolytic migratory erythema

Glucagonoma syndrome (diabetes mellitus, weight loss and anaemia) is associated with a characteristic skin rash (necrolytic migratory erythema) in 75% of cases. The lesion starts as an indurated erythematous area on the perineum, face and nose. Within a few days, blisters will cover the surface of the skin, which then crust and heal, leaving hyperpigmented skin. This process takes 7–14 days, with lesions developing in one area while others are resolving.

5.18   A: Excessive thyroxine is an additional risk factor for osteoporosis

Hyperthyroidism and excessive thyroxine treatment are secondary causes of osteoporosis. Plain X-rays are not sensitive enough to diagnose osteoporosis until total bone density has decreased by 30–50%. Results of bone mineral density (BMD) tests are typically reported as T-scores and Z-scores: the T-score compares a patient's BMD with the mean peak value for young, healthy adults of the same sex; the Z-score compares a patient's BMD with the mean value for people of the same age and sex. The World Health Organisation has defined osteoporosis as occurring when an individual's BMD is 2.5 standard deviations below the mean peak value in young normal adults. Hyperparathyroidism is another important cause of osteoporosis. It is associated with hypercalcaemia and low serum phosphate levels. All bisphosphonates act similarly on bone, by binding permanently to mineralised bone surfaces and inhibiting osteoclastic activity, thus inhibiting bone resorption, which means that less bone is degraded during the remodelling cycle.

5.19   E: Gigantism

Hypogonadism is a common feature in gigantism, leading to delayed epiphyseal closure and thus a more prolonged growth period. Klinefelter's syndrome is the most common cause of primary testicular failure and results in impairment of both spermatogenesis and testosterone production.

The other conditions listed are causes of precocious puberty, which is defined as the development of the menarche before the age of 8 years in girls or of secondary sexual characteristics before the age of 9 years in boys. It is accompanied by accelerated skeletal maturation and linear growth, with premature closure of the long bone epiphyses, resulting in short stature as an adult. Precocious puberty is classified into two types:

1   **True precocious puberty**, caused by premature secretion of gonadotrophins, which stimulate the production of testicular androgens and sperm. This results in virilisation and an increase in testicular size. Causes include:

  • idiopathic precocious puberty
  • central nervous system lesions which affect the posterior hypothalamus, eg craniopharyngioma, haematoma, hydrocephalus, neurofibroma, tuberous sclerosis, postencephalitic lesions
  • hCG-secreting tumours, eg hepatoblastoma
  • primary hypothyroidism, probably due to direct stimulation of FSH receptors by the high circulating levels of serum TSH; testicular enlargement and other features regress with thyroxine therapy.

2   **Precocious pseudopuberty** results from secretion of androgens from the adrenal gland or testes. Excessive androgens result in virilisation, but sperm production is not stimulated and the testes remain small. Causes include:

  • adrenocortical hyperfunction (congenital adrenal hyperplasia, virilising adrenocortical tumours
  • Leydig cell tumour
  • McCune–Albright syndrome (hyperpigmentation, polyostotic fibrous dysplasia, multinodular goitre and other glandular hyperfunction).

5.20   A: Zinc deficiency causes acrodermatitis and altered taste

Manganese deficiency causes dermatitis and nausea. Copper deficiency causes hypochromic microcytic anaemia, while excess copper in the circulation causes Wilson's disease. Chromium deficiency causes glucose intolerance. Zinc deficiency is also associated with poor wound healing.

5.21 C: Spontaneous recovery is expected in 90% of cases

Postpartum thyroiditis occurs in up to 5% of postpartum women, at least 3 months after delivery, and has two phases:

1 The **hyperthyroid phase** occurs alone in half of the cases with mild symptoms and may be associated with a small painless goitre. It can be differentiated from Graves' disease by the absence of thyroid-stimulating antibodies and low uptake of radioactive iodine. Antimicrosomal antibodies might be identified in 10% of cases but this does not help to differentiate between the two conditions.

2 The **hypothyroid phase** manifests 4–8 months after delivery and may or may not be preceded by a hyperthyroid phase.

5.22 B: Alcohol ingestion

The risk of coronary heart disease is inversely related to the level of high-density lipoprotein (HDL) cholesterol. HDL levels are significantly higher in women than in men at all ages. Levels are increased by regular exercise (eg jogging) and by the consumption of small amounts of alcohol. Levels are reduced in diabetes mellitus.

5.23 D: Try octreotide to control further hypoglycaemic attacks

Predisposing factors for severe sulphonylurea-induced hypoglycaemia include: advanced age; the use of long-acting agents, such as glibenclamide and chlorpropamide; and renal and hepatic disease. Sulphonylureas bind to receptors on β islet cells and this leads to insulin release. Fasting hypoglycaemia results if hyperinsulinaemia suppresses endogenous (predominantly hepatic) glucose production. Intravenous hypertonic glucose (20–50 ml 50% glucose via a large vein) will rapidly correct the hypoglycaemia but then acts as a potent secretagogue to the sulphonylurea-sensitised β cells. Insulin secretion is stimulated and hypoglycaemia recurs. Patients should be encouraged to take high doses of glucose orally once they regain consciousness. This will help to replenish the depleted glycogen stores in the liver.

Suppression of insulin secretion is a logical adjunct to intravenous glucose therapy in sulphonylurea-induced hypoglycaemia. The long-acting somatostatin analogue, octreotide has a potent inhibitory effect on insulin. Several reports have suggested that a combination of octreotide and dextrose should be considered for first-line treatment of sulphonylurea-induced hypoglycaemia. However, many authors prefer to reserve octreotide for more severe and resistant sulphonylurea-induced hypoglycaemia. Glucagon should be avoided as it stimulates insulin secretion. After good control of the hypoglycaemia has been achieved, which may take up to 72 hours of inpatient treatment, a shorter-acting oral hypoglycaemic drug such as gliclazide should be prescribed to replace the glibenclamide. The use of a long-acting insulin may lead to prolonged hypoglycaemia in patients with renal impairment.

5.24   A: Antiretroviral-related lipodystrophy

As the survival of HIV-positive patients improves, more complications of antiretroviral therapy are becoming apparent. These include a lipodystrophy-type syndrome characterised by the loss of peripheral and facial subcutaneous fat, but increased abdominal and visceral fat deposition. There is also an increase in the size of the dorsocervical fat pad – 'buffalo hump'. This fat redistribution is associated with a picture of abnormalities usually associated with insulin resistance, such as impaired glucose tolerance, low HDL cholesterol and high triglycerides. Glitazones may be of value in treating the condition, although some small trials have proved equivocal.

5.25   B: Wash out as many of his antihypertensive agents as possible for a period of 2 weeks, then review

The suspicion here, with hypokalaemia and metabolic alkalosis and resistant hypertension despite being on three agents, is that he has primary hyperaldosteronism. ACE inhibitors, angiotensin II-receptor blockers, diuretics, calcium-channel blockers and β-blockers all ideally require a wash-out period of 2 weeks to make the aldosterone : renin ratio assay meaningful; spironolactone requires a wash-out period of 6 weeks. A high aldosterone : renin ratio is suggestive of primary hyperaldosteronism. The blood sample should be taken in the morning, standing, and with a normalised potassium concentration (using supplementation) if possible. Urinary potassium excretion of >30 mmol/24 hours may be another useful clue in making the diagnosis.

Surgery is the treatment of choice for Conn's adenoma and leads to resolution of hypertension in around 70% of patients; mitotane may be useful for controlling the symptoms of adrenal carcinoma; and spironolactone is the medical treatment of choice for adrenal hyperplasia.

Chapter 6

GASTROENTEROLOGY

Answers

6.1   D: Cryptosporidiosis

Cryptosporidiosis is a parasitic protozoan infection that affects the gastrointestinal tract. The major symptoms are watery diarrhoea associated with cramping abdominal pain. Cryptosporidiosis occurs worldwide. Young children, the families of infected individuals, homosexual men, travellers, healthcare workers and people in close contact with animals comprise most reported cases. Oocysts may be identified by microscopy of faecal smears which have been treated with a modified acid-fast stain. The incubation period ranges from 1 day to 12 days, with an average of about 7 days. Patients may be infectious for as long as oocysts are excreted in the stool, from the onset of symptoms until several weeks after symptoms resolve. *Cryptosporidium* spp. are spread by the faecal–oral route, directly from person to person, from animal to person, or via contaminated food and water. Swimming pools are a common source of small outbreaks of cryptosporidiosis. Infected children are advised not to attend the swimming pool for 2 weeks after the diarrhoea has been controlled. The disease may sometimes be mild, but in people with impaired immunity, particularly those with AIDS, it may be a life-threatening illness.

Giardia infection is now recognised as one of the most common causes of water-borne disease. The organism is found in both drinking and recreational water and it is diagnosed by identifying *G. lamblia* trophozoites or cysts in the stool of infected patients. The standard stool ova and parasite (O&P) examination is usually used to identify *Giardia* cysts, rather than the modified acid-fast

189

stain. Amoebic dysentery (amoebiasis) is an infection of the intestine caused by *Entamoeba histolytica*, and usually affects people travelling in the tropics. The diagnosis is usually made by microscopic examination of the patient's stool specimen for *E. histolytica* trophozoites and/or cysts. Transmission of amoebic dysentery occurs mainly by ingestion of faeces-contaminated food or of water containing the *Entamoeba* cysts. The parasite or cyst does not survive long enough in the water of swimming pools to make these a source of an outbreak. *Staphylococcus* food poisoning and Norwalk virus gastroenteritis are not associated with cyst formation.

6.2   B: Crypt abscesses

Crohn's disease may involve any segment in the alimentary canal, but distal ileal involvement is characteristic. The inflammatory process involves all layers of the bowel, with the formation of non-caseating granulomas, ulcers and fistulae. Discontinuity of the inflammatory process, with 'skip lesions' along the bowel, is also characteristic.

In ulcerative colitis there is diffuse, continuous involvement of the colon, with proctitis as an early feature in 90% of cases. The inflammation is confined to the mucosa and lamina propria, with crypt abscess formation. Ileal involvement is not a common feature of ulcerative colitis, although the distal segment of the ileum can be involved in the inflammatory process from the adjacent inflamed colonic segment ('backwash ileitis').

6.3   D: Systemic mastocytosis in the stomach

Parietal-cell acid secretion is stimulated by one of the three principal mediators:

- gastrin
- acetylcholine
- histamine

Systemic mastocytosis is associated with high histamine production. Several hormones in the small intestine inhibit gastrin and gastric acid secretion in vivo. Resection of the small bowel leads to removal of this inhibition and hypersecretion of gastric acid results. Large-bowel resection has no effect on gastric acid secretion, however. In pernicious anaemia, gastrin levels are elevated in the presence of mucosal atrophy in the body of the stomach; acid production is therefore reduced. Steroid therapy and Cushing's syndrome have been associated with peptic ulcer disease, but it has not been demonstrated that this possible relationship is due to gastric acid hypersecretion. VIP inhibits gastric acid secretion and achlorhydria is a feature of VIP-secreting tumours.

6.4   D: It is caused by a Gram-positive anaerobic bacterium

Clostridium difficile, a Gram-positive anaerobic bacterium, is now recognised as the major causative agent of the colitis and diarrhoea that may occur following antibiotic intake. Infection with *C. difficile* represents one of the most common nosocomial (hospital) infections around the world. Diarrhoea is common in patients taking antibiotics (especially cephalosporins, ampicillin and clindamycin) but, in general, aminoglycosides are not known to cause the disorder. It is important to differentiate diarrhoea due to *C. difficile* (which may be life-threatening) from less serious, self-limited diarrhoea caused by antibiotics.

The symptoms vary from infrequent loose motions to severe watery diarrhoea with toxic megacolon. Bloody diarrhoea and abdominal tenderness are not features of pseudomembranous colitis and their presence suggests an alternative diagnosis. The sigmoidoscopic appearance of pseudomembranous colitis is diagnostic but not all patients demonstrate the lesions. As *C. difficile* may be present in the faeces of up to 20% of healthy carriers, the most specific test to determine if *C. difficile* is the cause of diarrhoea is the detection of toxins in faeces. Treatment consists of discontinuing the putative offending antibiotic agent and administering oral metronidazole, oral (rather than intravenous) vancomycin, or colestyramine. Clinical and laboratory predictors of positivity for toxin are the presence of faecal leucocytes (assessed by microscopy or lactoferrin assay), semi-formed (as opposed to watery) stools, the use of cephalosporins, and the onset of diarrhoea more than 6 days after the initiation of antibiotic therapy.

6.5   D: Intestinal lymphoma

Jejunal biopsy can be obtained by the blind suction technique (Crosby's capsule) or endoscopically. In coeliac disease there is total villous atrophy with elongated crypts and chronic inflammatory cell infiltration of the lamina propria. These findings are not specific, because they may occasionally be seen in other conditions, such as tropical sprue, bacterial overgrowth, lymphoma and Whipple's disease. However, in Whipple's disease the biopsy also demonstrates heavy infiltration of the mucosa by macrophages that stain positively with periodic acid-Schiff (PAS) reagent; the macrophages are filled with rod-shaped bacilli (*Tropheryma whippelii*). Endoscopy with biopsy is usually the diagnostic procedure of choice in intestinal lymphoma and eosinophilic gastroenteritis, in which there is infiltration of lymphocytes and eosinophils, respectively. *Giardia lamblia* flagellates attach to the mucosa of the duodenum and jejunum and cause inflammation and partial villous atrophy. Giardiasis is diagnosed by recognising the cysts in the stool (or sometimes flagellates in the jejunal fluid).

6.6   C: Mucosal dysplasia on colon biopsy is associated with the likelihood of carcinoma elsewhere in the bowel

The overall prevalence of cancer in all patients with ulcerative colitis is 3–5%. For those with pancolitis and disease duration greater than 10 years, the risk is 10–20 times greater than that of the general population. The prognosis of carcinoma of the colon developing in patients with ulcerative colitis tends to be worse than carcinoma developing in the absence of colitis because the diagnosis is often delayed because the symptoms of bleeding and diarrhoea may be attributed initially to a recurrence of colitis. The lesions are often multifocal and display a higher grade of malignancy. Carcinoembryonic antigen is not a reliable screening test for early colonic carcinoma. Colonoscopic surveillance programmes for colonic cancer are aimed at identifying mucosal dysplasia on biopsy specimens, which is associated with an increased likelihood of carcinoma elsewhere in the bowel.

6.7   A: Autoimmune hepatitis

This clinical picture and the liver function tests are typical of a patient with a chronic liver disease such as chronic active hepatitis (CAH). What differentiates autoimmune hepatitis from other types of CAH is the presence of autoantibody markers. A positive ANA, elevated IgG and positive anti-smooth muscle antibodies (ASMA) help to substantiate the diagnosis of autoimmune chronic active hepatitis. This is often divided in two subtypes, depending on the immune profile. Serum from patients with type 1 autoimmune hepatitis contains ANA and/or ASMA, whereas serum from patients with type 2 autoimmune hepatitis is positive for anti-liver-kidney-microsomal antibodies (anti-LKM1). Virtually all patients who are suspected of having autoimmune hepatitis should have a liver biopsy to confirm the diagnosis. Primary biliary cirrhosis and sclerosing cholangitis are diseases of middle-aged women. Antimitochondrial antibodies are characteristic of primary biliary cirrhosis. Gilbert's syndrome is not associated with significantly raised liver enzymes.

6.8   E: Solitary abscess in the right lobe of the liver

In developed countries, liver abscess (commonly of bacterial origin) usually complicates pre-existing biliary and gastrointestinal tract infections. Pyogenic liver abscess is caused by enteric flora (*Escherichia coli*, *Klebsiella* spp.) and *Staphylococcus aureus*. Unlike amoebic liver abscess, the symptoms are those of a systemic febrile illness lasting for days to weeks, and multiple abscesses are usually identified on ultrasound examination of the liver. Raised white cell count and other acute-phase reactants are common in both conditions. A solitary abscess in the right lobe of the liver is typical of amoebic liver abscess and these patients may give a history of chronic diarrhoea.

6.9   D: Anti-endomyseal antibodies

This patient has a malabsorption syndrome. The combination of iron deficiency anaemia and reduced serum folic acid levels indicates impaired absorption in the upper small intestine. Vitamin B12 is absorbed in the terminal ilium. A full blood count may reveal a microcytic anaemia due to iron deficiency or a macrocytic anaemia due to folate malabsorption; sometimes the picture is dimorphic.

Coeliac disease is a common cause of malabsorption. This is an inflammatory disease of the upper small intestine and results from gluten ingestion in genetically susceptible individuals. It is now estimated that coeliac disease may affect 1 in 200 people. Endomyseal antibodies are closely associated with gluten-sensitive disease, and in an appropriate clinical setting coeliac disease can be diagnosed with 100% specificity.

6.10   B: Carcinoid syndrome can manifest in the absence of liver metastases

Carcinoid tumours arise from enterochromaffin (Kulchitsky) cells that are located predominantly in the gastrointestinal mucosa. They are commonly found in the appendix or rectum. Clinical carcinoid syndrome is usually associated with carcinoid tumour that has spread to the liver. Tumours in sites such as the lung and the ovary can produce carcinoid syndrome without evident hepatic metastasis, however. Presumably, the liver clears mediators released from the tumour and this clearance is bypassed by liver metastases or when the tumour does not drain into the portal system. The syndrome is characterised by recurrent episodes of flushing, diarrhoea and hypotension. In long-standing cases, right-sided endocardial fibrosis, pulmonary artery stenosis, or tricuspid regurgitation might lead to progressive heart failure. Diagnosis is based on clinical suspicion and markedly elevated urinary 5-HIAA excretion. Chocolate, bananas and tomatoes may cause increased excretion of 5-HIAA.

6.11   C: Homozygous α_1-antitrypsin deficiency

Hepatocellular carcinoma usually complicates chronic liver disease secondary to alcoholic liver disease or viral hepatitis. Metabolic disorders which can be complicated by hepatocellular carcinoma include:

- haemochromatosis
- α_1-antitrypsin deficiency
- hereditary tyrosinosis
- glycogen storage disease type 1.

6.12   E: Gastrinoma

The clinical picture is that of multiple peptic ulcers and a pancreatic tumour. The most likely diagnosis is gastrinoma. Zollinger–Ellison syndrome (gastrinoma) is characterised by severe peptic ulcer disease and gastrin-secreting tumours of the pancreas. These gastrinomas generate high serum gastrin levels, leading to hypersecretion of gastric acid and consequent duodenal and jejunal ulcers. Gastrinoma should be considered in all patients with recurrent or refractory ulcer disease, ulcers associated with gastric hypertrophy, ulcers in the distal duodenum or jejunum, ulcers in association with diarrhoea, kidney stones, hypercalcaemia or pituitary disease, or in patients with a strong family history of duodenal ulcer disease or endocrine tumours.

Glucagonoma syndrome (diabetes mellitus, weight loss and anaemia) is caused by a hormone-secreting pancreatic tumour; peptic ulcer is not a recognised feature of the disorder. Although lymphomas are one of the common tumours of the bowel and may present with mucosal ulceration, the pancreas is not a particularly favourable site for lymphoma.

6.13   C: Hyperlipidaemia

Common causes of acute pancreatitis include alcoholism and biliary tract disease. Other causes include:

- trauma
- infections, eg coxsackievirus, mumps
- metabolic, eg hyperlipidaemia, hyperparathyroidism (but not hypoparathyroidism or diabetes mellitus)
- drugs, eg corticosteroids, azathioprine, thiazides, furosemide, phenformin, oral contraceptives, tetracycline
- systemic lupus erythematosus, polyarteritis nodosa (but not rheumatoid arthritis)
- familial.

6.14   A: This patient almost certainly suffers from chronic pancreatitis

Plain X-rays show pancreatic calcification in 25–59% of patients. This feature is pathognomonic for chronic pancreatitis. Chronic calcifying pancreatitis is invariably related to alcoholism. CT is excellent for imaging of the retroperitoneum, and it is useful in differentiating chronic pancreatitis from pancreatic carcinoma. The long history of pain and the presence of calcification go against a diagnosis of malignancy, however. Biopsy is not a standard test for chronic pancreatitis. Endoscopic ultrasound-guided fine-needle aspiration and cytology is used if pancreatic carcinoma is suspected. Endoscopic retrograde cholangiopancreatography (ERCP) provides the most accurate visualisation of the pancreatic ductal system and has been regarded as the standard method for diagnosing chronic pancreatitis. Excessive alcohol consumption is the most common cause, accounting for about 60% of all cases. Inherited pancreatitis and cystic fibrosis are other important causes of chronic pancreatitis. Gallstones play an important role in causing acute pancreatitis; they have no role in the aetiology of chronic pancreatitis.

6.15 A: Obesity

Fatty liver disease usually reflects excessive accumulation of triglycerides, which may be deposited either in large vacuoles that displace the nucleus or in small droplets with a central nucleus. Small fat droplets are usually associated with liver damage and abnormal liver function and carry a poor prognosis compared with the large vacuolar type of accumulation. Causes of fatty liver disease include:

1   Large fat globules (macrovesicular):

- obesity
- diabetes mellitus
- malnutrition
- corticosteroids
- ethanol ingestion.

2   Small fat droplets (microvesicular):

- acute fatty liver of pregnancy
- Reye's syndrome
- tetracycline
- sodium valproate
- ethanol ingestion.

Hypercholesterolaemia is not a condition known to cause fatty liver.

6.16   D: Colonoscopy

Gastointestinal blood loss should be considerd in men and postmenopausal women presenting with iron deficiency anaemia. When there is no obvious source of bleeding after thorough clinical assessment, you have to proceed to endoscopic investigation. Endoscopic examination offers the advantages of revealing a likely bleeding source in 80–95% of patients, allowing biopsy confirmation of some diagnoses, providing prognostic information and, often, permitting therapeutic intervention. Upper gastrointestinal bleeding is more common than lower gastrointestinal bleeding at this age and so oesophagogastroduodenoscopy (OGD) is performed as the initial test. For patients with lower gastrointestinal bleeding, sigmoidoscopy or colonoscopy is recommended to rule out specific pathology.

Barium meal is not a sensitive test and will not convey further information when the OGD is negative. Arteriography should be reserved for those patients with massive ongoing bleeding, when endoscopy is not feasible, or for patients with persistent or recurrent lower gastrointestinal bleeding in whom colonoscopy has not revealed a source. Bleeding from a small intestine source is very rare. Small-bowel barium enema is useful for identifying structural abnormalities such as strictures or space-occupying lesions; small bleeding lesions can easily be missed, however, and the yield is usually low.

6.17   D: Cholestasis of pregnancy may recur in a subsequent pregnancy

Viral hepatitis in pregnancy, particularly during the third trimester, appears to run a more severe course and is associated with an unusually high incidence of fulminant hepatic failure with high fetal and maternal mortality. Vertical transmission of hepatitis B virus infection occurs commonly when the mother contracts the disease during the third trimester. Acute fatty liver develops late in pregnancy, manifests initially with constitutional symptoms, often with abdominal pain, followed in many instances by hepatic failure with jaundice and encephalitis. The only known treatment is termination of pregnancy. It is not related to alcohol consumption. Cholestasis occurs late in pregnancy and is characterised by pruritus, sometimes followed by jaundice, which typically resolves within 2 weeks of delivery, but frequently recurs in subsequent pregnancies or with administration of contraceptives.

6.18   E: Sjögren's syndrome

The myriad causes of bilateral parotid swelling (other than mumps virus) include: infection with other viruses, such as parainfluenza virus type 3, coxsackieviruses and influenza A virus; metabolic diseases, such as diabetes mellitus and uraemia; and drugs, such as phenylbutazone and thiouracil. Other conditions associated with chronic parotid swelling include alcoholic liver disease, sarcoidosis, Sjögren's syndrome, lymphoma and HIV infection. Suppurative parotitis, usually caused by *Staphylococcus aureus*, is usually unilateral. Unilateral parotid swelling can result from a tumour, cyst or a ductal obstruction due to stones or strictures.

6.19   D: Diuretic therapy

The most likely explanation for this patient's recent deterioration is the development of hepatic encephalopathy. Hepatic encephalopathy may be precipitated by:

- deterioration in hepatic function
- drugs (sedatives, diuretics)
- gastrointestinal haemorrhage (usually with upper gastrointestinal bleeding – this leads to absorption of large amounts of protein and ammonia from the intestinal lumen)
- increased dietary proteins and constipation
- hypokalaemia
- infection
- azotaemia.

6.20   D: Gastric lymphoma

Consequences of *Helicobacter pylori* infection include duodenal and gastric ulcers and their complications, such as bleeding and perforation, atrophic gastritis, gastric cancer, and mucosa-associated lymphoid tissue (MALT) lymphoma. Epidemiological studies have shown that 95% of low-grade gastric MALT lymphomas are associated with *H. pylori* infection, and these lymphomas have been shown to arise from B-cell clones at the site of *H. pylori* gastritis. Eradication of *H. pylori* may lead to clinical and histological remission of these tumours in 70–80% of cases, but treated patients must be followed up closely for residual or recurrent lymphoma.

Patients with the varied group of upper gastrointestinal symptoms known as 'non-ulcer dyspepsia' may or may not be infected with *H. pylori*; at present, however, there is no generally recognised association between non-ulcer dyspepsia and *H. pylori* infection. Several mechanisms operate in the pathogenesis of reflux oesophagitis but there is no recognised association with *H. pylori* infection. More recently, it has also become evident that individuals without *H. pylori* are at greater risk for gastro-oesophageal reflux disease and its sequelae, Barrett's oesophagus and adenocarcinoma of the oesophagus. Achalasia of the cardia is a motility disorder leading to failure of relaxation of the lower end of the oesophagus and is not associated with *H. pylori* infection. Coeliac disease is a malabsorption syndrome caused by gluten sensitivity; it is an autoimmune disorder and is not associated with *H. pylori* infection.

6.21   B: In alcoholic hepatitis the AST : ALT ratio is 2 : 1

Alcoholic liver disease is the most common cause of cirrhosis in developed countries. Women are more susceptible to alcohol-related liver disease than men, even when consumption is corrected for body weight. Unlike viral hepatitis, alcoholic hepatitis is associated with a reversed AST : ALT ratio of 2 : 1. Alcoholic liver diseases include acute alcoholic hepatitis, chronic active hepatitis and alcoholic cirrhosis. Transferrin saturation and serum ferritin are commonly increased in alcoholic liver disease and minor degrees of iron overload are frequent. Alcoholic hepatitis and alcoholic fatty infiltration are reversible with abstinence and adequate nutrition.

6.22   D: Primary biliary cirrhosis

Primary biliary cirrhosis (PBC) should be suspected in a patient who reports unexplained itching and fatigue. The serum alkaline phosphatase concentration is invariably elevated in patients with PBC; almost all patients with PBC also have an elevated serum IgM concentration. If the alkaline phosphatase and serum IgM levels are both elevated and the antimitochondrial antibody test is positive, PBC is the most likely diagnosis. The diagnosis should be confirmed by percutaneous liver biopsy, which will show mononuclear inflammatory cells surrounding a small bile duct with proliferation and destruction of small bile ductules in the early stages, leading to fibrosis and cirrhosis in later stages. The diagnosis of PBC must be based on a combination of historical, laboratory, serological and histological criteria. In general, patients are middle-aged women who present with pruritus early and jaundice late. There is a recognised association between Sjögren's syndrome and autoimmune liver diseases such as autoimmune hepatitis and PBC.

6.23   C: Ureterosigmoid anastomosis

Certain chronic diseases of the colon predispose to cancer. In particular, long-standing ulcerative colitis and, to a lesser extent, Crohn's disease are associated with carcinomatous change. Conditions causing chronic inflammation, such as schistosomiasis, amoebic dysentery and tuberculosis, do not seem to predispose to cancer. Implantation of the ureters into the sigmoid colon predisposes to large-bowel neoplasia. Cholecystectomy may be associated with an increased risk of colorectal cancer, but the evidence is equivocal. Familial adenomatous polyposis is inherited as an autosomal dominant condition. Patients with familial adenomatous polyposis develop hundreds to thousands of colon polyps in adolescence and, if untreated, invariably develop colonic cancer by age 40; it accounts for only 1% of all colorectal cancers.

6.24   B: Chronic pancreatitis

This test distinguishes between malabsorption due to small-intestinal diseases and malabsorption due to pancreatic exocrine insufficiency. A 5-hour urinary excretion of 5 g or greater is normal following the oral administration of 25 g of D-xylose in a well-hydrated subject. Decreased xylose absorption and excretion are found in patients with damage to the proximal small intestine and in bacterial overgrowth in the small intestine (the bacteria catabolise the xylose). Patients with pancreatic steatorrhoea usually have normal xylose absorption. Abnormal results may be encountered in renal failure, in the elderly, and in patients with ascites caused by an excretion defect rather than by malabsorption.

6.25   E: Oesophageal varices

The liver receives approximately 1500 ml of blood each minute, two-thirds of which is provided by the portal vein. Portal hypertension is present when the wedged hepatic vein pressure is more than 5 mmHg higher than the inferior vena cava pressure. Because the veins in the portal system lack valves, increased resistance to flow at any point between the splanchnic venules and the heart will increase the pressure in all the vessels on the intestinal side of the obstruction. This is manifested clinically by the development of portosystemic collaterals (including oesophageal varices), splenomegaly, and/or ascites. Spider telangiectases, jaundice, hepatomegaly and gynaecomastia are manifestations of abnormal liver cell function.

Chapter 7

GENETICS

Answers

7.1   C: The limbs are short but the trunk height is normal

Achondroplasia is inherited as an autosomal dominant trait.
Approximately 80% of cases represent new mutations, the
mutation affecting endochondral ossification. The individual is
short in stature with short limbs (upper and lower limbs) but the
trunk is of relatively normal length. Complications include
hydrocephalus and spinal cord/root compression. Fertility and
intelligence are normal.

7.2   A: 47,XXY karyotype

Klinefelter's syndrome is a chromosomal abnormality and affected
individuals have a 47,XXY karyotype. Less than a third of patients
have gynaecomastia. In patients with primary hypogonadism the
testes are usually small (rarely exceeding 2 cm in length, the lower
limit of normal being 3.5 cm) and firm, this being due to fibrosis
and hyalinisation of the seminiferous tubules. Eunuchoid body
proportions, with tall stature and long legs are typical features. In
secondary (hypogonadotrophic) hypogonadism the testes are
small but soft. Other features of Klinefelter's syndrome include
azoospermia, testosterone deficiency and elevated gonadotrophin
levels.

**7.3   B: An alternative diagnosis should be considered if chorea
occurs in the absence of Kayser–Fleischer rings**

Wilson's disease is an autosomal recessive disease with a
prevalence of 1 in 30 000. Its clinical and pathological

manifestations result from excessive accumulation of copper in many tissues, including the brain, liver, cornea and kidneys. Impaired biliary copper excretion rather than enhanced absorption is the cause of the copper accumulation. Neurological manifestations typically appear between the ages of 12 and 30 years and are almost invariably accompanied by the presence of Kayser–Fleischer corneal rings. The amount of copper in the body at birth is normal. Evidence of haemolysis in patients with chronic liver disease is a clue to the diagnosis of Wilson's disease, but the haemolysis is not immune-mediated. Asymptomatic siblings who demonstrate biochemical evidence of the disease should receive treatment.

7.4   A: Huntington's disease

An autosomal dominant trait is one which is manifest in the heterozygote. Individuals affected with an autosomal dominant trait are usually found to have an affected parent. If an affected individual marries someone who does not have the disease and does not carry the affected gene, then, on average, half their children will develop the disease.

7.5   A: Sickle cell anaemia

Haemolytic anaemia may be congenital or acquired. Causes of congenital haemolytic anaemia include:

*   membrane defects, eg hereditary spherocytosis
*   enzyme defects, eg G6PD deficiency
*   haemoglobin defects, eg thalassaemia, sickle cell anaemia.

Sickle cell anaemia is caused by the inheritance of a gene for a structurally abnormal β-globin chain subunit of adult haemoglobin, HbS. The abnormal haemoglobin forms as a result of amino acid substitution in the polypeptide chains; the amino acid valine replaces glutamic acid at position 6 of the β-globin chain.

Beta-thalassaemia is caused by a failure in the synthesis of β chains. Hereditary spherocytosis and G6PD deficiency are not disorders of the β-globin chain. Methaemoglobinaemia results from NADH-methaemoglobin reductase deficiency, which causes the iron atom to be oxidized to the ferric form (Fe^{3+}), rendering the molecule incapable of binding an oxygen molecule. It causes persistent cyanosis without hypoxia, but does not cause haemolysis.

7.6   B: Leber's optic neuropathy

The prevalence of mitochondrial diseases is 1 in 10 000 liveborn infants. Mutation of mitochondrial DNA (mtDNA) is the most frequent cause. These diseases are often manifest as encephalomyelopathies, cardiomyopathies, vision disorders, dysacusis or metabolic disorders. Despite numerous studies, the mitochondrial diseases remain only partially understood. Leber's hereditary optic neuropathy was the first disease associated with hereditary point mutations in mtDNA to be described. The disease is characterised by subacute loss of binocular vision, with a lesion of the central field of vision, abnormal colour vision and atrophy of the optic nerve.

Another example of a mitochondrial disease is Kearns–Sayre syndrome, which is caused by both deletions and duplications of mtDNA. Symptoms of this syndrome appear before the age of 20 years, with short stature, pigmentary retinal degeneration, ophthalmoplegia, ptosis, ataxia, cardiac muscle conduction defects, diabetes and hearing loss. Chronic progressive external ophthalmoplegia (CPEO) is another mitochondrial disease. This may occasionally occur as a result of de novo mutation, may be maternally inherited (mt-tRNA mutations), or can have autosomal dominant inheritance. Symptoms of CPEO are ptosis, myopathy, depression, cataract and ketoacidosis. Alport's syndrome, Noonan's syndrome, Fabry's disease and Marfan's syndrome are diseases caused by mutations in nuclear and not mitochondrial DNA.

7.7   E: The diabetes mellitus is usually insulin-dependent

Idiopathic haemochromatosis is an autosomal recessive condition in which there is increased iron absorption in the gut. Clinically manifest hypogonadism is usually hypogonadotrophic in origin: iron deposition in the pituitary gland selectively inhibits gonadotrophin production without having any significant effect on the secretion of other pituitary hormones. The principal cause of death in patients with haemochromatosis is liver disease – hepatic failure and portal hypertension, and malignant hepatoma in 30% of cases. Another third of patients die of cardiac failure. Iron deposition in the renal parenchyma is of no clinical significance.

7.8   A: A heterozygous mother will transmit the trait to half of her daughters

A heterozygous mother will transmit the trait to half of her daughters. All daughters born to an affected father and a normal mother will be carriers. Half the daughters of a heterozygous mother will be carriers. Half of the maternal uncles will be affected. Heterozygous females occasionally exhibit mild features of the disease.

Chapter 8

HAEMATOLOGY

Answers

8.1 A: Philadelphia chromosome

In general, a leukaemoid reaction is a reflection of the response of healthy bone marrow to signals such as inflammation or infection; abnormally high white cell counts may be found in both these conditions. The combination of splenomegaly and a low alkaline phosphatase score would suggest CML as the likely diagnosis. The most definitive test, however, is a marrow chromosome analysis for the Philadelphia chromosome, which is pathognomonic for CML and is never found in leukaemoid reactions. More recently, DNA analysis showing *BCR* gene rearrangement has been found to be another useful marker for CML.

8.2 A: Hypersegmented neutrophils in the peripheral blood film

Hypersegmented neutrophils may appear in peripheral blood before there are signs of megaloblastic changes in the bone marrow: many neutrophils have more than four segments and occasionally they can have up to 16 segments. It is a very helpful finding and a reliable feature of megaloblastic anaemia. Giant metamyelocytes may be seen in the buffy coat of the blood, but megaloblasts are seen only in the bone marrow and are diagnostic.

Atrophic gastritis and achlorhydria are often present but are non-specific features. Intra- and extramedullary haemolysis occur to a substantial degree in megaloblastic anaemia, which leads to a raised LDH. This is an important clue to ongoing haemolysis, regardless of the cause. A low reticulocyte count and pancytopenia are features of bone marrow suppression of any cause. Although these are also features of megaloblastic anaemia, they are by no means specific.

8.3   D: Koilonychia is characteristic and is rarely seen in other forms of anaemia

Because of the large iron stores and the availability of iron in the average diet, iron deficiency caused solely by a poor diet is rare, even in women. Gastrointestinal bleeding is by far the most common cause of iron deficiency anaemia and is second only to menstrual loss as a cause in women. Spoon-shaped nails (koilonychia) are characteristic and are rarely described in other forms of anaemia. The spleen is slightly enlarged in 10% of cases. Paraesthesia in the absence of objective neurological findings may be seen in up to 30%, but this rarely progresses to peripheral neuropathy. The percentage and the absolute number of reticulocytes are both usually normal.

8.4   B: A monoclonal IgM peak

Waldenström's macroglobulinaemia is characterised by proliferation and accumulation of malignant cells with lymphoplasmacytoid morphology that secrete IgM. The clinical features include lymphadenopathy, hepatosplenomegaly and the hyperviscosity syndrome. Bone pain is not a feature of macroglobulinaemia and skeletal X-rays are usually unremarkable. In contrast to multiple myeloma, renal impairment and amyloidosis are quite rare. Other immunoglobulins (IgG, IgD) are commonly reduced.

8.5   B: Haemoglobin A_2 levels

A low mean corpuscular volume (MCV) and reduced haematocrit are found in both conditions. The peripheral blood smear is grossly abnormal in both thalassaemia trait and severe iron deficiency anaemia, both showing bizarre morphology, target cells and a small number of nucleated red blood cells. Splenomegaly is rare but may occur in 5–10% of patients with severe iron deficiency anaemia and in 5% of patients with thalassaemia trait. The haemoglobin A_2 level is elevated in thalassaemia trait; it is typically low in iron deficiency anaemia unless the patient has received a recent blood transfusion. Serum iron and ferritin levels are typically low in iron deficiency anaemia and high in thalassaemia trait.

8.6   C: Transfusion-related acute lung injury (TRALI)

Transfusion-related acute lung injury (TRALI) is manifest as the sudden development of severe respiratory distress and is caused by a syndrome of low-pressure pulmonary oedema resembling the adult respiratory distress syndrome (ARDS). These reactions are usually caused by the transfusion of antibodies in donor plasma that react with recipient granulocytes.

Leucocytes have increasingly been recognised as a contributor to, if not a cause of, a number of adverse reactions to blood transfusion. The major effects of donor leucocytes are either immunologically mediated or due to direct transmission of infection:

1   Immunologically mediated effects:

- febrile non-haemolytic transfusion reactions (FNHTRs) – the typical reaction consists of a chill followed by fever, usually during or within a few hours of the transfusion; headache and malaise may occur. Alloimmunisation to antigens on leucocytes and platelets is one of the most common causes of FNHTRs
- graft-versus-host disease (GVHD), which is the result of engraftment and proliferation of alloreactive donor lymphocytes in the transfusion recipient. Mature donor T lymphocytes detect alloantigens in the recipient and become activated, leading to inflammation and subsequent tissue damage. Skin rashes, fever, abnormalities of hepatic function, and diarrhoea occur; severe pancytopenia caused by marrow suppression is typical of transfusion-induced GVHD
- alloimmunisation against HLA – recipient antibodies react to HLA complexes on the platelet surface, leading to platelet destruction and shortened platelet lifespan. In patients who are refractory to platelet transfusion, HLA alloimmunisation is regarded as the main cause.

2   Infectious disease transmission, eg cytomegalovirus, Epstein–
Barr virus (EBV), human T-lymphotropic viruses 1 and 2
(HTLV-1 and -2).

8.7   A: Haemolytic anaemia associated with *Mycoplasma pneumoniae* infection

Therapeutic plasmapheresis is performed using a blood cell
separator to extract the patient's plasma, while returning the red
blood cells in a plasma-replacing fluid (eg 5% albumin).
Undesired plasma components are removed in this process, and
the remainder of the plasma is returned to the patient; a one-
volume exchange removes about 66% of such components.
Plasmapheresis may be used to supplement immunosuppressive
or cytotoxic therapy in the initial treatment of rapidly progressive
autoimmune processes. By rapidly removing undesired plasma
components (eg cold agglutinins, cryoglobulins and anti-
glomerular basement membrane antibodies), plasmapheresis
provides time for medications to exert their effects. Cold
agglutinins are circulating IgM antibodies that may increase in
response to certain infections, such as *Mycoplasma pneumoniae*
infections, and can result in cold agglutinin-mediated
autoimmune haemolytic anaemia. Plasmapheresis is very efficient
at removing big circulating molecules such as the pentameric IgM
molecules, in contrast to the relatively small, dimeric IgG
molecules. IgG-type antibodies are responsible for SLE-associated
haemolytic anaemia.

8.8   C: Acquired haemophilia

The acquired nature of this condition is invariably emphasised by
a negative distant past history of bleeding associated with
haemostatic challenges such as surgery. The most likely cause of
this patient's bleeding is acquired haemophilia. This is the term
used to describe the spontaneous development of inhibitors
(autoantibodies) to factors VIII or IX. Most patients present with
purpura, muscle bleeds and gastrointestinal bleeding, with no
previous history of bleeding disorder. Haemorrhagic
manifestations in patients with acquired haemophilia can be fatal
if not recognised and treated appropriately. Standard coagulation

studies show a normal prothrombin time (PT) and thrombin time (TT), and the platelet count and platelet function tests (including bleeding time) are normal. The APPT is prolonged, however. Specific factor assays will show a low level of factor VIII and detectable or high levels of factor VIII inhibitors.

Haemophilia is an X-linked disorder caused by a deficiency of factor VIII or factor IX coagulant activity. This disease manifests in young males. However, female carriers of severe haemophilia mutations frequently have reduced factor VIII or factor IX levels, which may predispose them to bleeding during invasive procedures or in the puerperium. Up to a third of haemophiliacs develop inhibitors in their blood. It rarely presents with spontaneous bleeding. Reduced factor VIII levels are also seen in inherited or acquired von Willebrand disease (vWD); platelet function and aggregation are often abnormal; and factor VIII inhibitors are absent. Bernard–Soulier syndrome is a platelet disorder and the partial thromboplastin time (PTT) is within the normal range. The PTT in disseminated intravascular coagulation (DIC) is prolonged but factor VIII levels are usually within normal limits and factor VIII inhibitors are absent.

8.9   E: It can transform to lymphoma

The cells of origin in the majority of patients with chronic lymphocytic leukaemia (CLL) are clonal B cells arrested in the B-cell differentiation pathway, intermediate between pre-B cells and mature B cells. CLL is characterised by the accumulation of small, mature B lymphocytes in the bone marrow and peripheral blood. About 1% of patients with morphological CLL express T-cell markers (CD4 and CD7) and have clonal rearrangements of their T-cell receptor genes. The presenting features are persistent lymphocytosis, lymphadenopathy and hepatosplenomegaly. The majority of patients live for 5–10 years, with an initial course that is relatively benign but followed by a terminal progressive and resistant phase lasting 1–2 years. The diagnosis is usually confirmed on peripheral blood examination; bone marrow examination is rarely required. Transformation of CLL to diffuse large-cell lymphoma (Richter's syndrome) carries a poor prognosis with a median survival of less than 1 year. Paraproteinaemia is a feature of plasma cell disorders and not of CLL. Furthermore, hypogammaglobulinaemia eventually develops in almost all patients with CLL, predisposing them to a number of infections, the most common being bacterial pneumonia.

8.10   E: Autoimmune haemolytic anaemia is a recognised association

Immune thrombocytopenic purpura (ITP) is thrombocytopenia occurring in the absence of toxic exposure or of other diseases associated with low platelets. The immune mechanism involves IgG-type antibodies. The disease is characterised by normal or increased marrow megakaryocytes, shortened platelet survival and the absence of splenomegaly. In neonatal ITP, IgG antibodies are transferred passively across the placenta: the infant platelet count may be normal at birth, but falls within 12–24 hours. It is rarely severe enough to result in bleeding diathesis in the infant. Evans' syndrome is a rare condition in which autoimmune haemolytic anaemia and thrombocytopenia occur in the same patient. Leukaemic transformation does not occur in ITP.

8.11   C: It results in a 'dry tap' marrow aspirate despite the presence of marrow hypercellularity

In hairy cell leukaemia (HCL), men are affected approximately four times more frequently than women. Anaemia and splenomegaly are the most common presenting features. Increased bone marrow reticulin often results in a 'dry tap' marrow aspirate despite the presence of hypercellularity. This, together with peripheral pancytopenia, might lead to an erroneous diagnosis of aplastic anaemia. Skin vasculitis (erythema nodosum, cutaneous nodules) occurs in as many as a third of patients.

8.12   C: The presence of Philadelphia chromosome

Good prognostic signs in ALL include:

*   FAB L1 type, cALLa
*   young age
*   pre-B phenotype
*   low initial white cell count.

Bad prognostic signs include:

- FAB L3 type
- Philadelphia chromosome
- central nervous system involvement
- T-cell type
- high initial white cell count.

8.13   B: Coeliac disease

Hyposplenism usually follows surgical removal of the spleen. Less often, hyposplenism is functional, when splenic tissue is replaced by abnormal tissue such as sarcoid granuloma, amyloid or myeloma protein. Other diseases linked to hyposplenism include coeliac disease, dermatitis herpetiformis, Graves' disease and systemic lupus erythematosus. Such patients run the same risk of fulminant bacterial infection as do those who have had their spleen surgically removed.The condition can often be diagnosed on peripheral blood smear examination: Howell–Jolly and Heinz bodies, nucleated red blood cells, siderocytes and acanthocytes are often seen.

8.14   A: Leucoerythroblastic blood picture

Myelofibrosis is a disease characterised by excessive fibroblast proliferation and collagen deposition in the bone marrow. It is accompanied by myeloid metaplasia and hypertrophy of organs such as the liver, spleen and lymph nodes. It is usually associated with a leucoerythroblastic blood picture, teardrop cells and poikilocytosis. It is a disease of the bone marrow and the bones are generally normal. It does not transform to multiple myeloma.

8.15   C: Factor VIII inhibitors occur in 10% of patients receiving multiple factor VIII transfusions

Petechiae are an extremely important clue in the diagnosis of haemostatic disorders and are only seen in platelet disorders. Haemarthroses are almost pathognomonic of severe haemophilia and often lead to joint damage and deformities. The bleeding in haemophilia is usually confined to soft tissue, muscle and other body compartments. The iron is usually recycled from these sites and iron deficiency anaemia is not a frequent feature of haemophilia. The partial thromboplastin time is prolonged; the prothrombin time and bleeding time are typically normal in haemophilia. A prolonged bleeding time is caused either by thrombocytopenia or by qualitative platelet dysfunction.

8.16   D: Iron deficiency anaemia due to blood loss

Thrombocytosis occurs in the following disorders:

- bleeding and haemolysis
- inflammation (rheumatoid arthritis, inflammatory bowel disease)
- post-splenectomy or functional hyposplenism (sickle cell disease)
- myeloproliferative disorders.

Pernicious anaemia and vitamin B12 deficiency lead to ineffective erythropoiesis associated with pancytopenia. The haemolytic-uraemic syndrome is characterised by microangiopathic haemolytic anaemia and thrombocytopenia. Paroxysmal nocturnal haemoglobinuria is often associated with aplastic anaemia. The antiphospholipid syndrome is a clinical disorder characterised by recurrent arterial and venous thrombotic events, pregnancy losses and/or thrombocytopenia. Thrombocytosis frequently occurs in association with iron deficiency anaemia, but the reason for this is not clear.

8.17   C: Human parvovirus B19 infection

Aplastic anaemic crises occur more frequently in children with a parvovirus infection, which is characterised by mild fever, dyspnoea on exertion, anorexia and pallor. Recovery from an aplastic crisis typically takes 1 week, but the patient may need to be transfused with packed erythrocytes until the marrow recovers. Well-known precipitants of vaso-occlusive pain crises (VPC) include cold weather, relatively high haemoglobin concentrations, dehydration, infection, exercise, dampness, poor diet, hypoxia, acidosis, emotional stress and fatigue.

8.18   E: Laboratory monitoring of activated partial thromboplastin (APPT) is not required

Both forms of heparin bind and activate antithrombin, accelerating the interaction of antithrombin with activated factor X (factor Xa) 1000-fold. After subcutaneous injection, LMW heparins are better absorbed and have higher bioavailability. The half-life of subcutaneous LMW heparin (3–6 hours) is two to four times that of unfractionated heparin. The risk of bleeding may be less with LMW heparin. Thrombocytopenia is induced by both types of heparin, but LMW heparin has a low affinity for platelet factor 4 and is therefore associated with a lower incidence than unfractionated heparin. Several clinical trials have shown that LMW heparins are at least as safe and effective as unfractionated heparin in the treatment of deep venous thrombosis.

LMW heparins have a longer half-life and a more predictable anticoagulant effect than unfractionated heparin, which allows for subcutaneous administration without laboratory monitoring. They exert their anticoagulant effect by inhibiting factor Xa but affect thrombin and factor IIa only minimally. The APTT, a measure of antithrombin (anti-factor IIa) activity, is not used to measure their activity; this has to be measured using a specific anti-Xa assay.

8.19   D: Thymoma

'Aplastic anaemia' comprises a diverse group of potentially severe marrow disorders which are characterised by pancytopenia and a marrow that is largely devoid of haemopoietic cells, which are replaced by a large amount of fat. Aplastic anaemia may be classified as constitutional or acquired.

Constitutional causes of aplastic anaemia include:

• familial or congenital
• Fanconi's anaemia
• dyskeratosis congenita.

Acquired causes of aplastic anaemia include:

• idiopathic (rarely associated with thymoma)
• autoimmune
• drugs, eg cytotoxic drugs, chloramphenicol, phenytoin, phenothiazines, thiouracil, methicillin

- toxic chemicals, eg benzene
- radiation
- pregnancy
- infections, eg hepatitis, parvovirus
- paroxysmal nocturnal haemoglobinuria.

8.20   C: The diagnosis can be made by assessment of serum ferritin level and liver biopsy

Chronically transfused patients inevitably develop a syndrome of iron overload called 'transfusion haemosiderosis'. However, only people who have received more than 100 units of packed erythrocytes (25 g of iron) develop symptoms of iron overload (similar to those observed in haemochromatosis). Desferrioxamine (Desferal®) is an effective and safe iron chelator. Pericarditis is the early and most frequent symptom of cardiac involvement. The diagnosis is made by assessment of the serum ferritin level and liver biopsy. Transfusion haemosiderosis develops more readily in thalassaemia than in aplastic anaemia.

8.21   C: Recombinant human erythropoietin (epoeitin)

The anaemia of chronic renal disease begins when the glomerular filtration rate falls below 30–35% of normal and is normochromic and normocytic. It is caused primarily by decreased production of erythropoietin by the failing kidney. Anaemia is often well tolerated in patients with chronic renal failure. This patient has ongoing ischaemic heart disease, which has been made worse by the anaemia resulting from his chronic renal failure. The patient is at higher risk for developing an acute cardiac event. Correction of the anaemia is mandatory to reduce this risk and to prevent recurrent anginal pain. Both the National Kidney Foundation and European best practice guidelines recommend evaluation of anaemia when the haemoglobin falls below 11 g/dl and consideration of treatment with recombinant human erythropoietin if the haemoglobin is consistently less than 11 g/dl, to maintain a target haemoglobin of over 11 g/dl. The haemoglobin should rise by 1–2 g/dl per month.

Iron, whether in oral or injectable form, is often recommended as an adjunct therapy to erythropoietin. Blood transfusion is used in more acute situations, when the anaemia is far more severe, or when the anaemia proves resistant to the above measures. B12 injection should only be considered if there is evidence of B12 deficiency, such as macrocytosis or low serum B12 concentration. Chronic renal failure is generally not associated with B12 deficiency or pernicious anaemia. Early investigations firmly established the stimulatory effects of androgens (nandrolone decanoate) on erythropoiesis, but their long-term use is associated with significant adverse effects. Once recombinant human erythropoietin became available, the use of these compounds was almost completely abandoned. Erythropoietin should be administered to pre-dialysis patients who have anaemia-dependent angina or severe anaemia with a haemoglobin concentration below 10 g/dl.

8.22   C: Spine

The sites most usually involved in bone metastasis are, in order of frequency, the spine, pelvis, ribs, skull and proximal long bones.

8.23   E: It is responsible for neural tube defects in the fetus

Reduced intake is by far the most common cause of folic acid deficiency. Because body folate reserves are small, deficiency develops rapidly (within 4 months) in people with an inadequate diet. Impaired utilisation of folate is caused by administration of methotrexate, a powerful inhibitor of dihydrofolate reductase that can deplete folate coenzymes in tissues within hours. Folinic acid rather than folic acid effectively counteracts the action of methotrexate by bypassing the inhibited reductase and is useful in the treatment of toxicity. Bacteria colonising the small intestine utilise vitamin B12 and generate folic acid. The lack of neurological findings in patients with megaloblastic anaemia suggests folic acid rather than B12 deficiency. Pregnancy increases requirements for folate. Folic acid supplementation is desirable during pregnancy, not only because requirements are increased but also because there is an increased risk of abruptio placenta, neural tube defects and spontaneous abortion in severe folic acid deficiency.

Chapter 9

INFECTIOUS DISEASES

Answers

9.1   E: Spontaneous bacterial peritonitis

Spontaneous bacterial peritonitis is an acute bacterial infection of ascitic fluid. Gram-negative enteric bacteria are the most commonly isolated pathogens: overall, *Escherichia coli*, *Klebsiella* spp. and *Streptococcus* spp. are responsible for 75% of all cases. Patients present with mild abdominal pain, anorexia and nausea, with or without fever, and leucocytosis, hypotension, and significant abdominal tenderness. Almost 33% of patients are essentially asymptomatic, however, and a slight change in mental status may be the only clinical evidence of infection. Any medical deterioration in a patient with cirrhosis and ascites should therefore prompt consideration of ascitic fluid infection. If untreated, it is associated with a high mortality. It was once thought that this condition was caused by transmural spread of bacteria, but it is now believed to be secondary to haematogenous spread in a host with depressed immune function.

Ascitic fluid leucocytosis, with an absolute count of more than 500 white cells/µl is the single best indicator of spontaneous bacterial peritonitis, being over 85% sensitive and 98% specific. As many as half the patients have negative routine ascitic fluid cultures, but these patients should be treated as aggressively as those with positive initial cultures. The treatment of choice is cefotaxime 2 g intravenously every 8 hours for 5 days.

9.2   C: Psittacosis ornithosis

The genus *Chlamydia* comprises two species, *C. psittaci* and

217

C. trachomatis. Chlamydia psittaci a ubiquitous cause of infection in birds and lower mammals, with humans as occasional accidental hosts, when it can cause serious pneumonic disease. *Chlamydia trachomatis* causes ocular infection (trachoma) which is regarded as the commonest cause of blindness in developing countries; *C. trachomatis* types L1, L2 and L3 cause proctocolitis and painful enlargement of the inguinal lymph glands (lymphogranuloma venereum). Reiter's syndrome is a disorder of unknown aetiology and is characterised by a triad of arthritis, conjunctivitis and urethritis; both *Chlamydia* and *Mycoplasma* organisms have been implicated in the post-venereal type.

Q fever is caused by *Coxiella burnetii*, a *Rickettsia*-like organism. The clinical features of the illness are protean, ranging from subclinical infection to fatal encephalitis and endocarditis. Chagas disease, named after the Brazilian physician, Carlos Chagas, who first described it in 1909, exists only in South and Central America. It is caused by a flagellate protozoan parasite, *Trypanosoma cruzi*. Lyme disease is caused by spirochaetal bacteria, *Borrelia burgdorferi*. River blindness (onchocerciasis) is an infection caused by the parasite *Onchocerca volvulus* (a worm) and is spread by the bite of an infected blackfly. It is called 'river blindness' because the transmission is most intense in remote African rural agricultural villages located near rapidly flowing streams.

9.3   B: Fragmented red blood cells are seen on peripheral blood film examination

Haemolytic-uraemic syndrome (HUS) is characterised by microangiopathic haemolytic anaemia and renal impairment that usually occur abruptly in children approximately 3–10 days after an episode of gastroenteritis or viral upper respiratory tract infection. Gastroenteritis is often associated with verotoxin; only 10% of cases progress to renal failure. *Escherichia coli* is not found in the blood at the time of diagnosis. Fever and neurological disorders are not characteristic features of HUS. The presence of these symptoms is more suggestive of thrombotic thrombocytopenic purpura. Complete recovery is expected in the majority of the cases. Fragmented red blood cells on peripheral blood film examination is a typical feature of microangiopathic haemolytic anaemia.

9.4   B: In *Plasmodium malariae* infection, a relapse can occur even 2 years after the patient has left an area prone to malaria

In *P. vivax* infection, fever and rigors usually manifest 2 weeks after an infected mosquito bite. Most *P. falciparum* infections are eliminated in 1 year; a few persist for up to 3 years. However, *P. malariae* infection, may persist as an asymptomatic infection for the life of the patient and a relapse can occur many years after an individual has left the malarial zone. Chloroquine is very effective for treating all types of malaria, including *P. falciparum* infection, but in certain areas in Asia and Africa *P. falciparum* is now chloroquine-resistant. Africans with sickle cell trait are often resistant to malarial infection. Malaria is diagnosed by identifying the parasites on thin and thick blood film examination.

9.5   A: *Staphylococcus epidermidis*

Bacterial infection of a prosthetic joint is a rare, but devastating and costly, event. Hip and knee replacements, which account for most of the joint replacement operations performed, have a 1–2% chance of becoming infected over the life of the patient or of the replacement.

The most common source of infection is seeding from an infected skin lesion, especially when infection occurs early, in the first 12 weeks (ie the postoperative period). Gram-positive staphylococci comprise 75–90% of the Gram-positive bacteria found in infected prosthetic joints, with *S. epidermidis* being more common than *S. aureus*, in contrast to septic arthritis in natural joints, when *S. aureus* predominates.

9.6   B: Hydatid disease

Hydatid disease is transmitted by accidental ingestion of the cyst of the parasite. The other disorders listed are arthropod-borne diseases (arthropods include lice, bed bugs, fleas, mosquitoes, ticks, mites etc):

- *Trypanosoma* is transmitted by tsetse flies
- leishmaniasis is transmitted by sandflies
- malaria is transmitted by mosquitoes
- Lyme disease is transmitted by ticks.

9.7   D: Resistance is most often encountered to isoniazid

Multidrug-resistant tuberculosis (MDR-TB) is caused by an isolate of *Mycobacterium tuberculosis* which is resistant to two or more of the first-line chemotherapeutic agents, usually isoniazid and rifampicin. There has been dramatic change in the epidemiology of TB since the description of AIDS in 1981. These changes include an increase in the number of primary TB cases reported and also an increase in MDR-TB cases. Sputum smear is positive for acid-fast bacilli in 70% of patients with MDR-TB, compared with 50% of patients with pan-sensitive organisms; this means that MDR-TB is more infectious. People who have been exposed to a case of MDR-TB, especially if they are immunocompromised, are at risk for developing MDR-TB. Other people who may develop drug-resistant tuberculosis include TB patients who have failed to take antituberculosis medications as prescribed, TB patients who have been prescribed an ineffective treatment regime and people who have been treated previously for TB. The resistance to isoniazid (the most common resistance to first-line drugs) is most commonly related to a change on the kat G gene (catalase/peroxidase).

Directly observed therapy is defined as observation of the patient by a health provider or other responsible person as the patient takes their anti-TB medication. So far, the most important ways of stopping the spread of MDR-TB are educating the TB patient to cover their mouth and nose when coughing, providing adequate treatment for people with MDR-TB, and providing directly observed administration of antituberculosis medications for people who are unwilling or unable to comply with prescribed drug plans.

9.8   B: Aciclovir

The clinical picture and the distribution of the rash is consistent with herpes zoster. Aciclovir has been shown to relieve and shorten the duration of the acute symptoms of herpes zoster as well as to shorten the duration of post-herpetic neuralgia. Antibiotics are not indicated unless there is evidence of secondary infection. Carbamazepine can relieve some forms of post-herpetic neuralgia, but the drug is not helpful for relief of acute zoster pain. A gluten-free diet is effective in the treatment of dermatitis herpetiformis (the distribution of the vesicular rash in this patient is not typical of this disorder). Cyclophosphamide is an alkylating agent used for the treatment of vasculitis and malignancies. The skin rash in this patient is not characteristic of a vasculitis.

9.9   A: Genital herpes

Infectious aetiologies of genital ulcers include herpes simplex virus (HSV), chancroid (*Haemophilus ducreyi*), granuloma inguinale (*Calymmatobacterium granulomatis*), syphilis (*Treponema pallidum*), HIV-specific ulcers (acute HIV infection or late HIV), and lymphogranuloma venereum (LGV, *Chlamydia trachomatis* serovars L1–3). Non-infectious aetiologies include fixed drug reactions, Behçet's disease, neoplasms and trauma. It is particularly important to consider these alternative causes if investigations for the infectious aetiologies do not lead to a diagnosis.

Genital ulcers occur in sexually active individuals throughout the world. The relative frequency of each of the infectious aetiologies differs depending on geographical location. The most common causes of genital ulcers in sexually active young adults in the USA are HSV, syphilis and chancroid. Of these three infections, ulcers due to HSV are the most prevalent, followed by primary syphilis and then chancroid. Infection with each of these organisms is not mutually exclusive, and co-infection with multiple organisms occurs. Genital ulcers caused by HSV are frequently multiple, shallow and tender, while chancroid often presents with deep, undermined and purulent ulcers. When a painless, indurated, clean-based ulcer is present, the diagnosis of syphilis is more likely.

There are a number of laboratory tests that can be used to make an accurate diagnosis. Conventional tests for diagnosing these infections include:

- Gram stain and culture on selective media (for *H. ducreyi*)
- Tzanck preparation, direct fluorescence antibody (DFA) and viral culture (for HSV)
- serological tests (for syphilis and LGV)
- dark-field microscopy (for syphilis, but not routinely available)
- tissue biopsy (syphilis, granuloma inguinale).

9.10   A: Meningococcal meningitis

Gram-staining should always be used in examining cerebrospinal fluid (CSF), as it permits rapid and accurate identification of the aetiological agent in approximately 60–90% of cases of bacterial meningitis. *Neisseria meningitidis* (meningococcus) is a Gram-negative diplococcus with flattened sides and a characteristic biscuit shape. Meningococcal meningitis can be caused by *N. meningitidis* groups A, B or C, or by other serogroups. Meningococci are confined entirely to humans; the natural habitat of these bacteria is the nasopharynx. The organisms are presumably transmitted from person to person through the inhalation of droplets of infected nasopharyngeal secretions and by direct or indirect oral contact. In non-epidemic periods, the overall rate of nasopharyngeal carriage is approximately 10% but may approach 60–80% in closed populations, such as those in military recruitment camps or schools.

Children under the age of 2 years have the highest incidence, with a second peak in the 15–24-year age group. In the UK there is currently an increased incidence of meningococcal disease among university students, especially among those in their first term who are living in catered accommodation.

9.11   A: *Pseudomonas aeruginosa*

Malignant external otitis is an infection of the external auditory canal caused by *Pseudomonas aeruginosa*, and is commonly seen in elderly patients with diabetes. The infection can spread from the outer ear to the soft tissues below the temporal bone and invade the parotid gland, temporomandibular joint, masseter muscle, and temporal bone. Necrotising osteitis of the temporal bone develops. The high mortality rate originally reported for the condition (approximately 40%) led to the use of the adjective 'malignant' for this form of temporal bone infection.

9.12   E: Hyponatraemia occurs significantly more often in Legionnaires' disease than in other pneumonias

Legionnaires' disease is sometimes overlooked as a possible cause of sporadic, community-acquired pneumonia. Water contaminated with the bacteria is the source of infection, and aspiration is the mode of transmission for most patients. High fever and gastrointestinal symptoms are clinical clues to this disease.

Legionella pneumophila is consistently ranked among the top three or four most common causes of community-acquired pneumonia; *Streptococcus pneumoniae* and *Haemophilus influenzae* are the two most common causes. Predisposing factors for Legionnaires' disease include age >50 years, cigarette smoking, and excessive alcohol intake. The risk of contracting Legionnaires' disease is unusually high in patients who have chronic lung disease and in those who are immunosuppressed. *Legionella pneumophila* is a Gram-negative rod and it is not readily seen on Gram stains of sputum. The urinary antigen test for *Legionella* species is most useful and should be available in every clinical microbiology laboratory. It is sensitive and highly specific. Results of this test can be available within hours after submission to the laboratory. The treatment of choice is macrolide or quinolone antibiotics.

9.13   A: The entire body can be checked for infectious disease sites

Indium leucocyte imaging (with ^{111}In-labelled leucocytes) is an isotope test in which the leucocytes which are tagged or labelled by the tracer in vitro are attracted to an inflammatory site. The test is useful for detecting occult abscesses and for screening the whole body in the search for a site of infection in patients with pyrexia of undetermined origin (PUO).

[111]In-labelled leucocyte imaging is useful for evaluating the activity of inflammatory bowel disease: although the scan cannot distinguish between the different causes of inflammatory bowel disease, it may be useful for showing the presence, distribution and extent of disease in a patient who cannot be subjected to more

invasive procedures. Recognition of a splenic abscess may be difficult because labelled leucocytes normally migrate to the spleen; gallium-67 (^{67}Ga) may be a better choice for spleen study because ^{67}Ga does not normally accumulate in the spleen. An RBC radioactive scan is usually used to determine a site of bleeding, particularly bleeding within the gastrointestinal tract.

9.14   A: The incidence of Kaposi's sarcoma in AIDS has been in progressive decline since the early 1990s

While the incidence of Kaposi's sarcoma (KS) as an AIDS-defining event has steadily declined from >30% in the mid-1980s to <15% by the mid-1990s, it remains the most common AIDS-related malignancy. With the advent of highly active antiretroviral therapy, the prevalence of KS and of other opportunistic infections and malignancies has dropped significantly over the past 5 years. It remains to be determined whether the incidence of KS will increase again as more patients fail antiretroviral therapy. Reports have documented that KS is ten times more common in homosexual and bisexual men than in heterosexual men infected with HIV. AIDS-related KS remains relatively uncommon among heterosexual intravenous drug abusers, women, and those acquiring HIV infections through blood products, suggesting a sexually transmitted agent has a causative role.

The importance of an altered immune system in the pathogenesis of KS is underscored by its 400× increased risk in organ transplant patients. As KS is not evenly distributed between all HIV risk groups and is rare among patients with congenital immune deficiencies, it is unlikely that immunosuppression is the sole aetiological factor. Several lines of epidemiological evidence suggest that the agent or agents involved in the pathogenesis of KS are sexually transmitted. Although AIDS-associated KS may involve any organ, mucocutaneous disease is the most common initial manifestation.

9.15   B: AIDS is the most likely diagnosis if *Mycobacterium avium-intracellulare* (MAI) is isolated from a biopsy specimen of an enlarged lymph node in an otherwise healthy individual presenting with generalised lymphadenopathy

Oral hairy leukoplakia is probably caused by Epstein–Barr virus (EBV). Because *Mycobacterium avium-intracellulare* (MAI) occurs so rarely in non-pulmonary tissue in association with any disease other than AIDS, its isolation from a lymph node in a previously healthy individual would strongly suggest the diagnosis of AIDS. Other causes of generalised lymphadenopathy include mononucleosis, toxoplasmosis, cytomegalovirus, syphilis and AIDS. Serology and lymph node biopsy are recommended for evaluation of patients with generalised lymphadenopathy.

Pneumocystis carinii derived from human specimens cannot be grown in vitro, nor is there a reliable serological test. To establish the diagnosis, the organism must be identified in pulmonary secretions or tissues. Cytomegalovirus infection is present in almost all AIDS patients and it is by far the most common cause of retinitis among these patients. For reasons that are not currently clear, Kaposi's sarcoma is almost never seen among AIDS patients who are not homosexual or bisexual.

9.16 B: Hypnozoites

It is important to know the details of the malaria life cycle. Hypnozoites represent the 'dormant' liver stage of the life cycle of *Plasmodium vivax* and *P. ovale* infection (ie benign malarias), and can cause late relapses after treatment. They are not part of the life cycle of *P. falciparum*. To eradicate hypnozoites and prevent such relapses, a course of primaquine must be given following chloroquine therapy for *P. vivax* and *P. ovale* infections. Primaquine is not required after quinine therapy for *P. falciparum* infection, but Fansidar® (pyrimethamine + sulfadoxine) or tetracycline are given to cover the possibility of low-grade quinine resistance.

9.17 B: Measles virus

The history is typical of measles, which has an incubation period of 8–12 days, followed by a 2–6-day prodrome with coryzal symptoms, conjunctivitis, dry cough and fever before the rash appears. Koplik's spots (small red lesions with a bluish-white centre on the buccal mucosa opposite the second molar teeth) appear during the prodrome. Rubella has a longer incubation period (12–21 days) than measles and is a milder illness, typically with a low-grade (or absent) fever and no significant respiratory symptoms (apart from coryza). Parvovirus B19 infection typically causes a 'slapped-cheek' appearance, but can mimic rubella. EBV is usually asymptomatic in young children, and mumps does not cause a rash.

9.18   B: *Staphylococcus aureus*

Important Gram-positive cocci include staphylococci, streptococci and enterococci. Staphylococci typically form clumps and clusters in culture, whereas streptococci characteristically grow in chains of variable length. *Staphylococcus aureus* is coagulase-positive, unlike *S. epidermidis*. *Enterobacter* spp. are Gram-negative coliforms – not to be confused with the Gram-positive enterococci, such as *E. faecalis* and *E. faecium*.

9.19   E: Yellow fever

Live vaccines, including rubella, measles, mumps, bacillus Calmette-Guérin (BCG), yellow fever and oral polio vaccine, are contraindicated in the immunocompromised. The hepatitis (formaldehyde-inactivated virus), typhoid Vi (polysaccharide antigen) and tetanus (adsorbed toxoid) vaccines pose no risk, although their efficacy may be reduced in the immunocompromised. Inactivated polio vaccine is available if needed (not the case here, as it is less than 10 years since her last booster), but polio has been eradicated in the Americas since 1991. Yellow fever vaccine is therefore the main problem.

9.20   A: Dysphagia

A diagnosis of chronic fatigue syndrome (CFS) requires the presence of unexplained chronic fatigue for more than 6 months. Although several formal definitions exist, cardinal features of CFS (besides fatigue) include impaired memory or concentration, sore throats, myalgia, arthralgia, headaches, unrefreshing sleep and post-exertion malaise. CFS is a diagnosis of exclusion, which requires the absence of any other underlying organic or psychiatric problems. Dysphagia is not a typical feature of CSF. Its presence in conjunction with general fatigue might reflect an underlying neuromuscular disorder and should be investigated urgently.

9.21 B: Interferon-α with ribavirin

Combination therapy with subcutaneous interferon-α (three times weekly) and oral ribavirin (daily) would be the most effective regimen of those in the list. Ribavirin alone has little or no effect. Lamivudine is licensed for the treatment of hepatitis B virus infection but not for HCV (it is also used in HIV therapy). New therapies for HCV are rapidly emerging, including pegylated interferons.

9.22 C: Cytomegalovirus (CMV) infection

The clinical picture and blood results are typical of CMV infection in the early post-transplant stage. In the first 6 months after a renal transplant, CMV is the responsible organism in two-thirds of febrile episodes. Patients present with fever, malaise, lymphadenopathy, arthralgias and myalgias, leukopenia with atypical lymphocytes, and mild elevations in liver transaminases. Many other organisms could present in similar fashion but they are not as prevalent as CMV in this patient group. Ganciclovir and valganciclovir are the standard treatment choices for this type of infection.

Acute rejection occurs within the first 3 months post-transplant: patients present with decreasing urine output, hypertension, rising creatinine levels and mild leucocytosis; fever, graft swelling, pain and tenderness may be observed with severe rejection episodes. Transplant-related (or acquired) Kaposi's sarcoma is 150 to 200 times more likely to develop in transplant patients than among the general population. Transplant-related Kaposi's sarcoma often affects only the skin, but in some patients the disease can spread to the mucous membranes or other organs. It usually presents as a red or brown skin nodule and is rarely associated with acute febrile illness.

9.23 C: Brucellosis

Brucellosis is a zoonotic infection that results from contact with farm animals (commonly sheep, goats, pigs, cattle or dogs). Most cases occur due to occupational exposure, for example in farmers, vets or abattoir workers. The most common infecting agents are *Brucella melitensis* and *Brucella abortus*. It is acquired via inhalation or ingestion of organisms or via a break in the skin. The incubation period is between 1 week and 3 months, with symptoms of fever, sweating, weight loss and mild depression. Hepatosplenomegaly is often present. Infection may rarely seed to heart valves, causing endocarditis, or to bone, resulting in osteomyelitis. The white cell count may be normal or low and the diagnosis may be confirmed by antibody testing. Combination treatment with doxycycline and rifampicin or with co-trimoxazole may be considered, and should be continued for 6 weeks or more; treatment courses of less than 6 weeks are associated with a significant relapse rate.

Chapter 10

NEPHROLOGY

Answers

10.1 E: Antithrombin III deficiency

Patients with nephrotic syndrome are at higher risk for developing arterial and venous thrombosis: the loss of antithrombin III and plasminogen via urine and the simultaneous increase in clotting factors, especially factors I, VII, VIII, and X, increase the risk. Renal vein thrombosis and pulmonary embolism are especially frequent. A low antithrombin III level (<75% of normal) and hypovolaemia are the major factors predisposing patients with nephrotic syndrome to arteriovenous thrombosis. All the other features mentioned in the list are factors associated with thrombophilia but do not play a major role in precipitating thrombosis in patients with nephrotic syndrome.

10.2 D: Primary membranous glomerulonephritis

Over 90% of patients with post-streptococcal glomerulonephritis have a reduced level of total haemolytic complement, or C3, with normal levels of C1q and C4, which suggests activation of the alternative pathway. Subacute bacterial endocarditis-associated glomerulonephritis is characterised by activation of both classical and alternative pathways; a similar picture often seen in shunt nephritis. Type 1 mesangiocapillary glomerulonephritis is associated with activation of the classical complement pathway, with depression of both C1q and C4. In SLE, the classical pathway is activated. Primary membranous glomerulonephritis and IgA nephropathy (Buerger's disease) are seldom associated with low levels of serum complement.

10.3   B: Almost all patients have ascites and are usually jaundiced

Hepatorenal syndrome describes the impairment in renal function that develops in patients with serious liver disease when all other causes of renal dysfunction have been excluded. The kidneys are normal histologically and the pathogenesis is unknown. There is intense intrarenal vasoconstriction and redistribution of blood flow. The liver disease is usually severe (patients are jaundiced) and almost all patients have ascites. The hallmark is oliguria and progressive decline in renal function. The urine is typically free of protein or any other sediment. Uraemia may develop and may be treated with dialysis. If the liver disease improves, normal renal function returns. The prognosis is poor, with over 80% of patients dying during hospitalisation from liver failure or complications of portal hypertension.

10.4   B: Bilateral small kidneys

When a patient presents for the first time with renal impairment it is very important to identify the duration of renal failure, as it will influence the management and prognosis. Anaemia, hypocalcaemia and dilute urine can be encountered in both acute and chronic renal failure. Acute pulmonary oedema and seizures are a consequence of volume overload in both acute and chronic renal failure. Bilateral small kidneys on imaging and evidence of renal osteodystrophy on plain X-ray reflect long-standing pathology more suggestive of chronic renal failure. Skin pigmentation and peripheral neuropathy may also result from long-standing metabolic abnormalities such as chronic renal failure.

10.5   C: Microscopic polyangiitis

Microscopic polyangiitis is the most common cause of the pulmonary-renal syndrome: approximately 90% of patients have glomerulonephritis. Equally common is renal involvement in Wegener's granulomatosis: 80% of patients will go on to have glomerulonephritis. Compared with these two vasculitides, the other common vasculitis syndromes involve much less frequent and less severe renal disease. Inflammatory renal artery stenosis with hypertension is encountered in some patients with Takayasu's arteritis.

10.6   C: Linear deposits at the glomerular basement membrane on indirect immunofluorescent testing

Goodpasture's syndrome is a disease of young males (6 : 1 male to female ratio) and is characterised by a triad of pulmonary haemorrhage, glomerulonephritis and anti-glomerular basement membrane antibody (anti-GBM) production. There is a characteristic, continuous, linear pattern of IgG deposition along the capillary wall. The disease usually begins with pulmonary haemorrhage, which is manifest as haemoptysis, dyspnoea and pulmonary alveolar infiltrates seen on X-ray, and iron deficiency anaemia. The pulmonary symptoms are followed within days to weeks by the development of haematuria and proteinuria and by a rapid loss of renal function. There is no documented specific skin rash. Although all the features mentioned in the list are typical of Goodpasture's syndrome, the most characteristic feature is the histopathological appearance.

10.7   A: Low back pain is the most common presenting symptom

Retroperitoneal fibrosis is one of a group of multifocal fibrosclerotic syndromes, which also includes mediastinal fibrosis, sclerosing cholangitis and Riedel's thyroiditis. The process usually begins over the promontory of the sacrum and extends laterally across the ureters and as high as the second or the third lumbar vertebrae. It is more common in men (2 : 1) and the peak incidence is in the fifth and sixth decades. Low back pain is the most common symptom, which may be accompanied by fever and weight loss. Methysergide, a $5HT_2$-antagonist used to treat migraine headache, can cause a similar syndrome; other drugs, such as β-blockers, methyldopa and hydralazine have also been implicated. Pizotifen is an antihistamine; its use is not associated with retroperitoneal fibrosis. Systemic diseases associated with retroperitoneal fibrosis include systemic lupus erythematosus, scleroderma and carcinoid syndrome. The diagnosis is suggested by the finding of displacement of the ureters towards the midline during intravenous pyelography. The fibrosing process may surround the inferior vena cava, but obstruction of that vessel is uncommon. Thromboembolism and hypertension are recognised complications. The fibrous tissue does not infiltrate the kidneys or the ovaries.

10.8   E: Hyperplasia of the juxtaglomerular apparatus

Bartter's syndrome is a childhood disease which has an autosomal recessive inheritance. The pathophysiology of the disease is thought to be due to impaired loop sodium chloride reabsorption, which causes increased renin and aldosterone secretion with juxtaglomerular hyperplasia. Enhanced sodium chloride delivery to the collecting duct stimulates potassium secretion, leading to hypokalaemia. It also causes hydrogen ion secretion, resulting in metabolic alkalosis. Accelerated kinin and prostaglandin secretion may account for the vascular unresponsiveness to pressor effects. This explains the absence of an increase in blood pressure and oedema, despite the elevated levels of renin and aldosterone. Indometacin inhibits prostaglandin and restores the normal physiological vascular response.

10.9   A: Amyloidosis

Other causes of impaired renal function and enlarged kidneys include:

* stage 1 diabetic nephropathy
* hydronephrosis
* acromegaly
* renal vein thrombosis.

10.10 B: Active urinary sediment with red blood cell casts indicates glomerulonephritis

Henoch–Schönlein purpura (HSP) is a systemic small-vessel vasculitis which mainly involves the blood vessels of the skin, gastrointestinal tract, kidneys and joints. HSP mainly affects children between the ages of 3 years and 10 years and boys are affected more often than girls (3 : 2). In approximately two-thirds of children, an upper respiratory tract infection precedes the onset of HSP by 1–3 weeks. The hallmark of the disease is the characteristic palpable purpura, which is seen in nearly all patients. It is caused by inflammation of dermal blood vessels and not by thrombocytopenia. Apart from raised circulating IgA, the immunology profile, including pANCA and the anti-glomerular basement membrane antibody test, is usually negative.

HSP nephritis becomes clinically manifest in only 20–30% of cases. It usually presents as macroscopic haematuria and proteinuria, lasting for days to weeks. Most glomeruli look normal under light microscopy, with only a few showing mesangial proliferation. The most consistent finding is deposits of IgA in the mesangium; focal and segmental intracapillary and extracapillary proliferation with adhesions in small crescents is sometimes seen. Granuloma formation is not a feature of HSP.

10.11 A: Plasma osmolality

Both conditions are associated with polyuria (excessive urine production) and polydipsia (excessive thirst). In both conditions, the urine specific gravity is 1.005 or less and the urine osmolality is less than 200 mosmol/kg. However, a low plasma osmolality (<285 mosmol/kg) with a history of psychiatric disease is highly suggestive of psychogenic polydipsia. In diabetes insipidus the plasma osmolality is generally slightly higher (290–300 mosmol/kg).

An MRI scan of the pituitary is mandatory after central diabetes insipidus has been confirmed using a water deprivation test. Ultrasound of the kidneys has no place in the investigation of polyuria/polydipsia disorders. Patients with chronic renal failure describe polyuria, but almost all these patients have abnormal renal function and renal ultrasound will not add any further information, apart from showing small kidneys and so confirming an already established cause of polyuria or polydipsia.

Psychogenic polydipsia is usually a late manifestation of schizophrenia, occurring in 10–40% of such patients (who hold an irrational belief that drinking water is healthy – thirst is not given as a reason for drinking). It may also occur in the manic phase of bipolar disorders (usually transiently). Although a psychiatric assessment might reveal an underlying psychotic disorder, which will suggest the diagnosis, it would not be useful for establishing the cause of polyuria with any certainty.

10.12 C: Aciclovir

Due to poor solubility in urine and associated dehydration, certain drugs can lead to crystal deposition in the tubules and collecting ducts in the kidneys. This will lead to obstruction, which may present as acute renal failure. Aciclovir is rapidly excreted in urine, especially after bolus intravenous therapy. Birefringent needle-shaped crystals can be seen in the urine, particularly using polarised light.

Sulfadiazine and sulfamethoxazole (but not penicillins) are now being used in higher than usual doses to treat toxoplasmosis in patients with AIDS and can cause crystal deposition in acidic urine. The most common forms of crystals are needle-shaped and rosettes. The ingestion of ethylene glycol or, rarely, high doses of vitamin C can result in acute renal failure due to the overproduction and deposition of oxalate crystals. Allopurinol lowers serum uric acid levels by inhibiting the conversion of hypoxanthine and xanthine to uric acid: hypoxanthine and xanthine are water-soluble and readily excreted in urine with no tendency for crystal or stone formation. ACE inhibitors and gentamicin cause renal disease but not through crystal deposition.

10.13   C: Granular casts are often associated with renal parenchymal disease

Hyaline casts are seen in normal individuals and their identification in a urine sample carries no special clinical significance. The presence of fat globules on urine microscopy indicates significant proteinuria and probably nephrotic syndrome. A finding of dysmorphic red blood cells points towards a glomerular disease. Green urine colour may be due to urinary tract infection caused by *Pseudomonas aeruginosa* (not *E. coli*).

10.14   C: Dysequilibrium syndrome

These symptoms are typical of dysequilibrium syndrome. This is caused by cerebral oedema, resulting from rapid shifts of uraemic toxins associated with too-rapid haemodialysis in a severely uraemic patient.

The symptoms of air embolism depend on the position of the patient. In a recumbent patient, air inside the heart impairs cardiac performance. In an upright position, the cerebral vessels are obstructed, resulting in central nervous system symptoms.

Fortunately, air embolism is extremely uncommon. Dialysis against a hypotonic dialysate is another extremely rare complication, as modern dialysis machines have on-line monitoring of dialysate conductivity; the features of this condition are those of severe intravascular haemolysis, with lumbar pain, hyperkalaemia and cerebral oedema.

Pericardial tamponade most commonly occurs in a patient who has severe uraemia causing pericarditis and impaired coagulation. The heparinisation which is a feature of conventional haemodialysis then causes haemopericardium. This patient would be at risk of haemopericardium, but the clinical features are not typical. Patients who are receiving rapid ultrafiltration (water removal) are at risk of intravascular volume contraction, manifest by hypotension. The elderly and those on antihypertensive drugs are at greatest risk, but the projected fluid losses in this patient are modest.

10.15 D: A deletion on the short arm of chromosome 11

Wilms' tumour is a disease of childhood, which makes an environmental aetiology (especially smoking!) less likely than genetic factors. There are several syndromes associated with Wilms' tumour, such as the AGR triad (aniridia, ambiguous genitalia and mental retardation). They are all associated with deletions on the short arm of chromosome 11.

Renal cell carcinoma is associated with cadmium exposure, lead toxicity, and smoking. Transitional cell carcinomata are associated with smoking, β-naphthylamine, Balkan nephropathy, analgesic nephropathy and schistosomiasis.

10.16 E: Multiple *café au lait* spots and subcutaneous nodules

The *café au lait* spots and subcutaneous nodules would suggest that he has neurofibromatosis, which is associated with renal artery stenosis (and also, incidentally, with phaeochromocytoma). Wheezing, flushing and diarrhoea may indicate carcinoid syndrome, which is not associated with renal pathology. Cushing's syndrome, Conn's syndrome and polycythaemia rubra vera are associated with hypertension but not with renal artery disease.

10.17 E: Renal involvement

The presence and severity of renal involvement in this patient are indicators of poor prognosis. Older patients also tend to fare less well, usually as a result of infective complications of treatment. Alveolar haemorrhage is a poor prognostic sign, as it is the cause of the majority of deaths in patients with the condition. However, the presence of extrarenal vasculitis is not thought to be indicative of a poor prognosis; indeed, some studies suggest it may place patients into a good prognostic group. The presence of cANCA, although a useful aid to diagnosis, is not a prognostic indicator.

Factors influencing the renal prognosis includes the proportion of sclerosed glomeruli found on renal biopsy, as well as the degree of interstitial scarring and atrophy. However, a high proportion of active crescents is not a prognostic indicator. The initial response to therapy (within 2 weeks) is a useful prognostic indicator.

10.18 B: Haematuria

There is reduced renal reabsorption of glucose in pregnancy, which may cause glycosuria, but patients with persistent glycosuria should be investigated with a glucose tolerance test at around 24 weeks. Ketonuria may also be seen in a normal pregnancy; it occurs as a result of the increased metabolic requirements. Early in pregnancy, the plasma osmolality falls by an average of 10 mosmol/kg. This is principally due to hyponatraemia: the osmotic thresholds for antidiuretic hormone (ADH) release are reduced, so that ADH is not suppressed. Dilatation of the renal pelvises and ureters is seen in 90% of women by the third trimester. Other physiological changes in pregnancy include: increased creatinine clearance; reduction in plasma uric acid (by 25% in the first trimester); decreased potassium excretion; hypercalciuria; and mild proteinuria (up to 500 mg/24 hours). Haematuria is not a feature of normal pregnancy and further investigation is warranted to identify an underlying renal problem or other pathology.

10.19 B: Diverticulitis

The most common cause of acute peritonitis in peritoneal dialysis (PD) patients is primary peritonitis, which is due to contamination of the PD fluid or catheter with skin organisms such as coagulase-negative staphylococci or *Staphylococcus aureus*. The presence of mixed Gram-negative and/or anaerobic organisms is highly suggestive of secondary peritonitis due to a perforated large bowel or appendicitis. Diverticulitis is the most frequent cause of this presentation. Other clues to the presence of intra-abdominal pathology are slow resolution of peritonitis, air under the diaphragm on a plain abdominal X-ray (although this may occur during the course of normal PD) and elevated PD fluid amylase. It is essential to examine the hernial orifices carefully to look for evidence of strangulated hernia. The outcome of secondary peritonitis is much worse than that of primary peritonitis, primarily because of the delay in diagnosis.

10.20 C: Rhabdomyolysis

Rhabdomyolysis occurs after extensive blunt trauma, such as that occurring after a motorcycle accident. Diagnosis is made by the presence of myoglobin on dipstick urinalysis (shows as haematuria), raised serum creatine kinase levels, hyperkalaemia, hypocalcaemia, hyperphosphataemia and hyperuricaemia. Aggressive intravenous fluid replacement is required to prevent acute renal failure, which may occur in up to 30% of cases of rhabdomyolysis. The rise in creatine kinase levels is detectable a few hours after injury and peaks at about 48 hours.

Rhabdomyolysis is also common after electrical injury, compartment syndrome, prolonged limb or tourniquet anaesthesia, extensive surgical dissection, and in infectious or inflammatory myopathies.

Chapter 11

NEUROLOGY

Answers

11.1 D: Observe in hospital and delay lumbar puncture and CSF analysis until the next morning

The classic presentation in cases of subarachnoid haemorrhage (SAH) is sudden onset of headache, frequently described as the worst ever experienced. There may be transient loss of consciousness or focal neurological deficit, and a history of associated vomiting is often given. The guidelines state that when the clinical presentation suggests SAH, computed tomography (CT) of the brain should be performed, and that when CT is negative or equivocal, then cerebrospinal fluid (CSF) should be examined. Xanthochromia, detected either visually or by spectrophotometry, where available, avoids the pitfalls of the traumatic tap: it becomes detectable between 6 and 12 hours after the onset of headache (it is preferable to delay the lumbar puncture until 12 hours after the onset of headache to avoid the possibility of a false-negative result). A CT scan of the brain is far more sensitive soon after the onset of SAH. Repeat CT brain scan is not necessary. MRI studies of the brain offer no further information in patients with suspected SAH who have a normal CT brain scan.

11.2 C: Thymoma on CT scan of the chest

Myasthenia gravis is an acquired autoimmune disorder associated with acetylcholine receptor deficiency at the motor end plate. Ocular muscle involvement is usually bilateral, asymmetrical and typically associated with ptosis and diplopia. Pupillary and accommodation reflexes are characteristically normal. Two-thirds of patients with myasthenia gravis have thymic hyperplasia and 10–15% will have thymoma. The creatine kinase is typically normal. Exophthalmos (proptosis) and diplopia are suggestive of

Graves' disease, in which there is restriction in upward and/or outward gaze – this is due to swelling and fibrosis of the inferior rectus and inferior oblique muscles beneath the globe rather than to weakness of the superior eye muscles.

11.3   A: Double vision on looking upwards

Cavernous sinus thrombosis is usually due to a suppurative process in the orbit, nasal sinuses or upper half of the face and is usually caused by *Staphylococcus aureus* infection. The condition is severe and associated with high fever, headache, malaise, nausea, vomiting and convulsions. Chemosis, oedema and cyanosis of the upper face occur due to obstruction of the ophthalmic vein. Ophthalmoplegia is secondary to damage to the IIIrd, IVth and VIth cranial nerves. Eye pain and hyperaesthesia of the forehead (not the chin) is caused by damage to the first division of the trigeminal nerve. Retinal haemorrhage and papilloedema are late events. Visual acuity may be normal or mildly impaired. Neither the facial nerve nor the lower cranial nerves pass through the cavernous sinus.

11.4   A: The trauma to the head is usually minor and often forgotten by the patient

The clinical syndrome may develop weeks or even months after the original trauma. The minor head injury might not be remembered by the patient. Headache is the earliest feature and may be present almost from the time of the injury; subsequently, subtle mental changes may occur, such as lethargy, loss of initiative, somnolence and even confusion. If untreated, patients may progress to develop the symptoms and signs of tentorial herniation. The bleeding is from cerebral veins. Lumbar puncture should be avoided because of the potential risk of tentorial herniation. Neck stiffness is a feature of arachnoid mater irritation due to subarachnoid haemorrhage.

11.5   B: Dura mater

Pain-sensitive structures within the central nervous system include:

- dura mater
- Vth, IXth and Xth cranial nerves
- blood vessels.

Other brain structures are not particularly sensitive to painful stimuli due to the paucity of pain-sensitive nerve endings in these structures.

11.6   B: Absent ankle jerk

Vitamin B12 deficiency causes degeneration of the white matter in the dorsal and lateral columns of the spinal cord, peripheral nerves, optic nerves and cerebral hemispheres. Multiple sclerosis (MS) is a demyelinating disease, in which the loss of myelin sheath also occurs primarily in the white matter of the brain, spinal cord and optic nerves. Neurological manifestations of vitamin B12 deficiency include a sensory peripheral neuropathy, with absent distal tendon reflexes and distal sensory loss. As the illness progresses, subacute combined degeneration of the cord develops and the patient may develop a Babinski sign and sensory ataxia. Pyramidal signs, cerebellar ataxia and pallor of the optic disc are also common features of MS, but sensory loss consistent with peripheral neuropathy is not a feature. Barber's chair sign (an electric shock-like sensation on forward bending of the head) is most commonly due to MS but is not diagnostic because it may occur with other lesions of the cervical cord, such as cord compression, syringomyelia and vitamin B12 deficiency.

11.7   D: It has a strong familial tendency

Essential tremor manifests as tremor of the hand, the head and, least commonly, the voice. Compared with Parkinson's tremor, it is more rapid and occurs on volitional movement. It is not associated with rigidity or hypokinesia. It is suppressed by alcohol and β-blockers. There is a strong family history and the incidence is distributed as an autosomal dominant trait. Though it manifests in the elderly, the age of onset varies and it can start as mild tremor in the third decade and worsen with advancing age.

11.8   B: Foot drop

The sciatic nerve originates in the sacral plexus, mainly from the

L5–S2 spinal segment. It supplies muscles that cause extension of the thigh and flexion of the leg. It divides into two major branches, the tibial nerve and the common peroneal nerve, which are responsible for all foot movements. Anterior thigh and medial leg sensory loss is typical of a femoral nerve lesion. The femoral nerve mediates flexion of the hip.

11.9 B: Lewy bodies

The characteristic microscopic finding in Parkinson's disease is the Lewy body. A cytoplasmic inclusion, the eosinophilic Lewy body typically consists of a dense core surrounded by a less intensely stained region and a faint halo. The peripheral halo of the Lewy body is composed of neurofilaments that stain for tau and ubiquitin. Lewy bodies have been identified in other disorders (corticobasal ganglionic degeneration and diffuse Lewy body disease). In addition, Lewy bodies have been noted incidentally during postmortem examination of elderly patients, with an increasing prevalence in patients aged 60 and older. The significance of this finding is unclear, although a preclinical form of Parkinson's disease has been suggested as the cause.

11.10 A: Wilson's disease

'Chorea' refers to brief, involuntary, irregular, non-rhythmic, non-repetitive semi-purposeful movement and manifests as 'milkmaid' grip, an inability to keep the tongue protruded, a stuttering gait and clumsiness, with a tendency to drop objects. Common causes of chorea include:

- hereditary, eg Huntington's disease, Wilson's disease, ataxia telangiectasia
- infections, eg Sydenham's chorea, encephalitis
- drugs, eg L-dopa, oestrogen, phenytoin
- metabolic and endocrine, eg chorea gravidarum, thyrotoxicosis
- vascular, eg lupus erythematosus, polycythaemia rubra vera

Haemochromatosis as such is not associated with chorea. However, many end-stage liver disorders may manifest with extrapyramidal signs. Motor neurone disease is associated with lower motor neurone lesion signs with fasciculations. Multiple myeloma and salbutamol therapy are not associated with chorea.

11.11 A: Shy–Drager syndrome

Autonomic neuropathy is commonly associated with other forms of neuropathy. It can be asymptomatic or it can cause incapacitating disability. There are three types of autonomic dysfunction:

1   Gastrointestinal:

- gastroparesis
- episodic nocturnal diarrhoea
- colonic dilatation.

2   Cardiovascular:

- postural hypotension
- elevated heart rate
- loss of respiratory sinus arrhythmia.

3   Genitourinary:

- large residual volume
- retrograde ejaculation
- impotence.

Autonomic neuropathy may be a manifestation of either a central or a peripheral nervous system abnormality:

1   Central nervous system:

- primary selective autonomic failure (Shy–Drager syndrome)
- Parkinson's disease
- Wernicke's encephalopathy
- syringomyelia/syringobulbia.

2   Peripheral nervous system:

- familial dysautonomia (Riley–Day syndrome)
- familial amyloidosis
- Guillain–Barré syndrome
- diabetes mellitus
- tabes dorsalis

- alcoholic nutritional neuropathy
- Eaton–Lambert syndrome (but not myasthenia gravis).

Vitamin B12 deficiency, multiple sclerosis and dermatomyositis are not associated with autonomic neuropathy.

11.12 D: Multiple sclerosis

This patient exhibits multifocal neurological dysfunction involving the optic nerve, cerebellum and spinal cord. The neurological symptoms have developed at different times during the period of her illness. The magnetic resonance imaging (MRI) revealed evidence of discrete lesions in the white matter. The whole picture is highly suggestive of multiple sclerosis. Syringomyelia and amyotrophic lateral sclerosis are not associated with specific brain abnormalities on MRI scan. Secondary brain metastases are usually associated with multiple lesions, but often there is prominent interstitial oedema surrounding the lesions, with or without tissue or midline shift. Multiple cerebral infarcts often affect both the grey and the white matter of the brain, unlike multiple sclerosis, in which the pathological process of demyelination is confined exclusively to the white matter where the myelin sheaths are found.

11.13 C: There is a bilateral Babinski sign

Syringomyelia is a disorder characterised by slowly progressive enlargement of a fluid-filled cyst, or 'syrinx' within the cord or medulla oblongata. It can cause damage to the anterior horn cells, the crossing of the spinothalamic tract fibres and the lateral corticospinal tract at the cervical or thoracic level. The clinical features include muscular weakness in the hand and arms, scoliosis, loss of arm reflexes, and spastic weakness with bilateral upgoing toes in the lower limbs. There is 'dissociated sensory loss', in which there is impaired perception of pain and temperature with preserved light touch perception and proprioception in the neck, arms and upper trunk. Extension into the medulla oblongata may cause nystagmus, dysphagia, or wasting of the tongue. Some patients have hydrocephalus or cerebellar signs related to an associated congenital craniocervical malformation (Chiari malformation).

11.14 E: Cluster headache

These are classic features of cluster headache. Cluster headache afflicts less than one in a thousand in the general population. The majority of sufferers are men. The syndrome is characterised by frequent attacks of intense pain localised in and around the eye on one side, characteristically accompanied by conjunctival injection and lacrimation in this eye, along with nasal stuffiness on the same side and sometimes Horner's syndrome. All signs and symptoms are strictly unilateral and only occur during attacks, which last for between 15 minutes and 3 hours. The attacks can occur from one to eight times a day, during a period lasting from some weeks to months. After a remission of varying duration, the same pattern recurs. In contrast to patients with migraine, patients with cluster headache prefer to pace about during an attack. Attacks frequently occur at night. Recent findings suggest a pivotal role of the hypothalamus in the pathophysiology. Sumatriptan injection or oxygen inhalation aborts pain attacks in most patients. The most frequently used prophylactic agents are verapamil, lithium and steroids. The long history makes headache due to brain tumour unlikely in this patient.

11.15 B: Posterior cerebral artery

Ipsilateral IIIrd nerve palsy with contralateral hemiplegia (Weber's syndrome) is the result of interruption of the posterior cerebral artery blood supply to the cerebral peduncle and the midbrain tegmentum.

11.16 B: Visual-evoked potentials (VEPs)

The clinical picture is highly suggestive of multiple lesions in the central nervous system and spinal cord. Also, the presence of transient phenomena in the past (the leg symptoms) makes a demyelinating disorder the most likely diagnosis. Visual-evoked potentials (VEPs) are cerebral potentials evoked by visual stimuli (a flash or black-and-white checkerboard pattern) and detected by scalp electrodes placed over the occiput. The method is highly sensitive for detecting demyelination of the optic nerve and central visual pathways. In multiple sclerosis, VEPs may demonstrate abnormality when the magnetic resonance image is normal, because optic nerve involvement often occurs early and may be asymptomatic.

11.17 A: Small irregular pupil

This patient's presentation is typical of sensory ataxia. The patient may be partially compensating for sensory ataxia using visual clues. For this reason, the patient will complain that inco-ordination is worse in the dark or when the eyes are covered, for example when dressing. The 'wash-basin sign', (falling or imbalance when splashing water on the face) and loss of balance when passing a towel over the face or pulling a shirt over the head are characteristic features of sensory ataxia. Patients often have a 'stamping' gait. This usually indicates a lesion in the dorsal columns of the spinal cord, with impaired proprioception. Romberg's test is a simple and sensitive bedside test that points to sensory ataxia as the cause in a patient presenting with postural imbalance.

Sensory ataxia should be differentiated from cerebellar (nystagmus), frontal lobe (grasp reflex) and vestibular ataxia. When weakness is present, it makes all assessment tests for ataxia invalid and may lead to false-positive results, so normal muscle power should be established before any attempt is made to examine for ataxia. Pill-rolling tremor is a feature of Parkinson's disease and, though associated with poor gait and posture, is not associated with dorsal column disease or sensory ataxia. Weakness and muscle fasciculation are classic features of motor neurone disease, which is not associated with dorsal column lesions.

Tabes dorsalis is regarded as the classic cause of sensory ataxia and therefore the small irregular pupil (Argyll Robertson pupil) is a very significant finding in this patient. Other causes of sensory ataxia include B12 deficiency, diabetes mellitus and other hereditary ataxias.

11.18 B: Creutzfeldt–Jakob disease

Prion diseases are fatal neurological disorders associated with the accumulation within the central nervous system (CNS) of insoluble aggregates of modified cell membrane protein called 'prion' protein. Only four human diseases have been associated with the accumulation of prion protein in the CNS: kuru, Creutzfeldt–Jakob disease, fatal familial insomnia and Gerstmann–Straussler disease.

11.19 D: Multiple sclerosis

Normally, cerebrospinal fluid (CSF) gamma-globulin comprises less than 13% of total CSF protein. The gamma-globulin is mostly IgG, but often contains IgA and IgM. Discrete oligoclonal bands in the gamma-globulin region are seen in 90% of patients with multiple sclerosis. Other conditions associated with a similar CSF finding include subacute sclerosing panencephalitis, chronic meningitis, neurosyphilis, and any condition that causes peripheral paraproteinaemia (such as multiple myeloma). Myasthenia gravis is a disease of the neuromuscular junction and is not associated with any changes in the CSF.

11.20 B: Cerebrospinal fluid (CSF) rhinorrhoea is a recognised presenting feature

The clinical features and computed tomography scan findings are suggestive of empty sella syndrome. In this syndrome the sella turcica is enlarged and filled with CSF. The pituitary gland is flattened along the posterior part of the floor. The aetiology is unknown, but the syndrome has been postulated to be due to incomplete formation of the diaphragma sella, permitting CSF pressure to be transmitted to the sella and gradually leading to herniation of the arachnoid and remodelling of the sella. Nearly all patients are asymptomatic, though some may have non-specific headache. The syndrome is more common in obese multiparous women and is associated with systemic hypertension and CSF rhinorrhoea. Endocrine function is generally normal, though there may be diminished thyroid-stimulating hormone and gonadotrophin secretion. The CSF pressure is usually normal.

11.21 A: Benign intracranial hypertension (BIH)

Benign intracranial hypertension (BIH), also known as 'pseudotumour cerebri', is a syndrome of increased intracranial pressure which is not associated with localising neurological signs, an intracranial mass lesion, or with cerebrospinal fluid outflow obstruction, in an alert, otherwise healthy-looking patient. The causal mechanism is unknown. Although it may present as asymptomatic papilloedema, most patients complain of headache, with or without nausea and vomiting. Bilateral papilloedema, the cardinal feature, is almost invariably present and may be associated with haemorrhages, exudates or both. Visual loss, the only serious complication of BIH, may occur early in the course of the disease. The lumbar spinal fluid pressure is usually elevated, frequently above 300 mmH$_2$O (hence the name of the condition). Diplopia, caused by unilateral or bilateral VIth (abducent) nerve palsy, may develop as a false localising sign.

Disorders associated with BIH include:

- endocrine disorders, eg Addison's disease, Cushing's syndrome, obesity, steroid therapy/withdrawal
- drugs, eg nalidixic acid, phenytoin, tetracycline, vitamin A
- haematological disorders (cryoglobulinaemia, iron deficiency anaemia).

Hydrocephalus (canal obstruction) is usually associated with dilated lateral ventricles. Subdural haematoma is uncommon at this age and usually evident on computed tomography brain examination. The long-standing history of headache goes against a diagnosis of subarachnoid haemorrhage.

11.22 E: Segmental demyelination on nerve conduction studies

Inflammatory demyelinating polyradiculoneuropathy often affects proximal rather than distal limb muscles. The most striking findings on examination are diffuse weakness and widespread loss of reflexes. Cerebrospinal fluid (CSF) protein peaks in the second or third week of the illness. Nerve conduction studies typically shows gross reduction in conduction velocities consistent with segmental demyelination. CSF cells and serum creatine kinase are typically within normal limits. Incontinence of urine is not a feature of Guillain–Barré syndrome.

11.23 C: Carotid artery dissection

Cervical carotid artery dissection is a significant cause of stroke in patients under the age of 40. The three most common presenting features are headache, contralateral transient ischaemic attack (TIA) and/or stroke, and ipsilateral Horner's syndrome (miosis, ptosis and facial anhidrosis). Internal carotid artery dissection usually occurs extracranially (ie in the neck). It occurs in previously healthy individuals and develops either spontaneously or following various degrees of trauma. Dissections are usually subadventitial (between the media and adventitia or within the media), creating a false lumen that can cause stenosis, occlusion, or pseudoaneurysm of the vessel. Simultaneously, the dissection may cause the formation of a thrombus, from which fragments embolise. Strokes resulting from carotid dissection can therefore have either a haemodynamic or an embolic aetiology. Horner's syndrome is present in approximately 50% of presenting patients and is probably due to the sudden enlargement of the internal carotid artery, which stretches or compresses the sympathetic fibres. An interesting feature is that headache usually precedes a cerebral ischaemic event, unlike a headache associated with stroke, which usually follows or accompanies the ischaemic event.

Temporal arteritis is extremely rare in patients under 50. It is associated with sudden visual loss due to ischaemic optic neuritis. It is not associated with Horner's syndrome. Myasthenia gravis is not associated with pupil abnormalities. Posterior communicating artery aneurysm is associated with an isolated IIIrd cranial nerve palsy; ptosis and a dilated pupil are the standard features. Pancoast tumour is an apical carcinoma of the bronchus which is often associated with local invasion of adjacent structures, including the sympathetic chain, causing an isolated ipsilateral Horner's syndrome. It is not associated with a concomitant cerebrovascular accident.

11.24 B: Pregnancy has no ill effects on the course of the disease

Multiple sclerosis is a disorder of unknown aetiology, defined by its clinical features and by the typical scattered areas of brain, optic nerve and spinal cord demyelination. It has a remitting and relapsing course. It is almost unknown in oriental people and among black Africans. Migrants from a high- to a low-prevalence area have a reduced risk of developing the disease, though this is true only for those who move before the age of 15 years. Elevation of body temperature by as little as 0.5 °C noticeably worsens the neurological deficit in some patients. This is the result of slowed axonal conduction induced by heat. Pregnancy has no ill effects on the course of the disease. Bad prognostic indicators include male gender, young age, incomplete recovery from the initial attack, and recurrent relapses with short recovery periods; motor, brainstem, and cerebellar dysfunction at the outset of the disease are also associated with a relatively poor outcome. Recently, interferon-α has been found to be helpful in selected cases. Facial nerve palsy is not a recognised feature of multiple sclerosis.

11.25 A: Temporal lobe haematoma with brain swelling

He has focal signs, with dysconjugate gaze. This indicates that a structural cause is more likely than a diffuse metabolic cause (although it should be remembered that focal signs can also occur in metabolic coma). In this case the history of a very sudden dramatic loss of consciousness, rather than a gradual deterioration, also points to a 'structural' rather than to a metabolic cause. The signs are those of a right IIIrd nerve palsy and, as such, are most likely to be due to downward compression of the IIIrd nerve by supratentorial pressure ('coning'). Pontine lesions tend to produce bilateral pinpoint pupils.

Chapter 12

OPHTHALMOLOGY

Answers

12.1 C: Central scotoma on perimetry

Optic neuritis is a demyelinating disease of the optic nerve head which is characterised by acute pain behind the eyes, particularly on moving the eyes, and with rapid deterioration of the central vision (central scotoma). The changes are difficult to differentiate from papilloedema on examination of the retina. Enlargement of the blind spot and, later, the development of tunnel vision are characteristic of papilloedema. Both conditions can be associated with slurred speech, diplopia, hemianopia or limb weakness; these features are related to the underlying cause.

12.2 D: A 74-year-old man with multiple cholesterol emboli on fundoscopy

A branch retinal artery occlusion can lead to an altitudinal field defect with visual loss in either the upper or lower visual fields. Fundoscopy may demonstrate embolic material within blood vessels. Anterior ischaemic neuropathy due to vasculitis of the posterior ciliary arteries usually causes altitudinal visual loss. Denial of blindness due to lack of awareness of the visual loss is a recognised feature of cortical blindness. Macular degeneration is associated with central scotoma and loss of central vision in the affected eye. Swelling of the optic disc due to papilloedema is often associated with tunnel vision. Acromegaly is typically associated with bitemporal hemianopia.

12.3 E: Ocular myasthenia gravis

The patient has signs attributable to reduced function of the lateral rectus, levator palpebrae superioris, inferior rectus and superior oblique muscles. He has retained normal function of the inferior oblique and superior rectus muscles, however. These signs are not compatible with a single lesion: a lesion of the superior branch of the IIIrd cranial nerve, for example, would be expected to affect both the levator and the superior rectus muscles.

12.4 B: Photophobia on ophthalmoscopy

Enteropathic arthropathy and other spondyloarthropathies are associated with iritis, which is characterised by ocular injection, photophobia, miosis (due to ciliary spasm), normal or near-normal visual acuity and a normal fundus. Conjunctivitis causes a purulent discharge and is irritable but not painful.

12.5 E: Carotid Doppler

Episodic total loss of vision in one eye is called 'amaurosis fugax'. In the majority of cases this is due to ipsilateral carotid artery disease. The lack of a bruit does not exclude severe stenosis, and the investigation of choice is a carotid Doppler. Rarer causes of amaurosis fugax include hyperviscosity syndromes, atrial fibrillation and valvular heart disease.

12.6 D: Proteinuria

The Wisconsin Epidemiological Study showed that the incidence of macular oedema was 2–6% in background retinopathy, 20–63% in preproliferative retinopathy, and 70–74% in proliferative retinopathy. The prevalence increased with the duration of diabetes and with higher glycosylated haemoglobin and proteinuria levels.

12.7 A: Posterior communicating artery aneurysm

The IIIrd (oculomotor) nerve emerges in the interpeduncular fossa, passes between the posterior cerebral and superior cerebellar arteries and pierces the dura at the lateral clinoid process to enter the lateral wall of the cavernous sinus. Causes of palsy include posterior communicating artery aneurysm, pressure on the nerve in coning, and diabetes: aneurysm is more commonly associated with headache; coning and the resulting IIIrd nerve palsy often develop gradually over many hours; and the palsy associated with diabetes is usually painless (and is, incidentally, associated with sparing of the pupillomotor fibres). Ophthalmoplegic migraine is a much less common cause of a painful IIIrd nerve palsy and should be a diagnosis of exclusion.

12.8   E: Retrobulbar neuritis

As the optic discs appear normal, and given the transient nature of her previous symptoms (which occurred during exam-time), it may be tempting to pass off the alleged blurring as factitious. However, in retrobulbar neuritis it is said that 'the patient sees nothing and the doctor sees nothing'. As the inflammation is behind the optic nerve head (hence 'retrobulbar'), as opposed to optic neuritis, the optic nerve head or optic disc appears normal. Optic nerve function, however, is affected in the same way in patients with optic and retrobulbar neuritis. The visual acuity will therefore be reduced to a very variable degree, and an afferent pupillary defect will be apparent during the 'swinging flashlight test'. Colour vision will be reduced to a greater extent than might be predicted from the visual acuity: red desaturation – when red looks paler to one eye than to the other – is a sensitive sign of optic nerve dysfunction. Visual field defects will occur (typically a central scotoma, but the type of defect varies). Retrobulbar neuritis has the same systemic implications as optic neuritis, in that an episode of optic or retrobulbar neuritis can contribute to a diagnosis of multiple sclerosis, if other neurological episodes separated in time and site occur.

Holmes–Adie pupil is an idiopathic condition, typically affecting young women, and presents with an enlarged pupil that is poorly reactive to light and accommodation. Absent ankle jerks are a frequent association. A Holmes–Adie pupil causes no problems, except for blurring of vision when reading in some patients. Parinaud's syndrome is caused by a lesion in the dorsal midbrain, and causes a variety of signs, including mid-dilated pupils, upper lid retraction and paralysis of upward gaze.

12.9   D: Retinitis pigmentosa

The combination of heart block, ocular myopathy and pigmentary retinopathy is known as Kearns–Sayre syndrome. This mitochondrial cytopathy occurs sporadically. The patients may also have short stature, ptosis, deafness, dementia and raised cerebrospinal fluid protein levels. Patients with ocular myopathy have limited eye movements but usually no diplopia because the eyes are involved symmetrically.

12.10 C: Giant-cell infiltrate in a temporal artery biopsy

This is the strongest evidence and should always be sought when long-term steroid therapy is contemplated. The normal erythrocyte sedimentation rate (ESR) is the age + 10 divided by 2 for females, and age divided by 2 for males. An ESR of 40 mm/hour is therefore normal for this lady. The C-reactive protein level may be abnormal but this has many causes.

Chapter 13

PSYCHIATRY

Answers

13.1 B: The hiccups stop when she is asleep

Hiccups are defined as recurring, unpredictable, clonic contractions of the diaphragm which produce sharp inhalations. Persistence of hiccups during sleep suggests an organic cause; if the hiccups stop during sleep and recur promptly on awakening, this would suggest psychogenic hiccups. Around 92% of cases of psychogenic hiccups occur in women; in men, the cause of the hiccups is often organic. Hiccup results from stimulation of one or both limbs of the hiccup reflux arc (the vagus and phrenic nerves, with a 'hiccup centre' located in the upper spinal cord). Organic causes of hiccups include central nervous system, upper gastrointestinal and diaphragmatic disorders.

Hiccups are a common disorder and fortunately are usually transient and benign. For every self-limiting disease, there are always many effective cures. Most of these cures work through stimulation of the glossopharyngeal nerve. Breath-holding and the Valsalva manoeuvre might help to abort these attacks but do not help to discriminate between psychogenic and organic causes. Major tranquillisers and metoclopromide are used in resistant cases. The response to these drugs is variable and not particularly unique to organic or psychological causes of hiccups.

13.2 D: Grasp reflex

Somatic complaints, such as anorexia, weight loss and headache, are features of both conditions, though more prominent in patients with depression. Behavioural and cognitive functions are affected in both conditions. Poor concentration, poor attention span, poor memory and social withdrawal are encountered in both. A grasp reflex and other primitive reflexes indicate neuronal loss in the frontal lobe, which does not occur in depression. A positive response to antidepressant treatment would be a reliable sign in favour of a diagnosis of depression.

13.3 C: A 50-year-old man with a history of suicide attempts

A variety of factors are associated with an increased risk of suicide:

1 Psychiatric disorder: psychiatric illness is the strongest predictor of suicide. The most commoly associated psychiatric disorders are depression, alcoholism and personality disorders.
2 History of previous suicide attempts or threats: patients with a prior history of suicide attempts are five to six times more likely to make another attempt; up to 50% of successful suicides have made a prior attempt.
3 Age and sex: the risk of suicide increases with increasing age. It is more common in the elderly. Women attempt suicide four times more frequently than men, but men are successful three times more often.
4 Marital status: the risk is higher in people who have never been married, widowed or separated.

Other factors include unemployment, chronic painful conditions, terminally ill patients and those who live alone. HIV infection alone does not appear to increase the risk of suicide.

13.4 D: The disorder may follow group A β-haemolytic streptococcal pharyngitis

Obsessive–compulsive disorder (OCD) is a common major mental disorder. It is characterised by anxiety-provoking intrusive thoughts and repetitive behaviours. Obsessions may consist of aggressive thoughts and impulses, or fears of contamination by germs or dirt; compulsions, such as washing, checking or counting, are rituals whose purpose is to neutralise or reverse the fears. Unlike thought insertion, which is one of the cardinal features of schizophrenia, obsessive thoughts are produced by one's own mind rather than inserted by anyone else or by an outside influence, and are perceived as senseless and intrusive into conscious awareness. Feelings of guilt are suggestive of depression, although depression can develop secondary to OCD. The thoughts and acts in OCD are not inherently pleasurable and are unpleasantly repetitive and the patient has often made unsuccessful attempts to resist them.

One of the most recent developments is the identification of a paediatric subgroup of patients with OCD, characterised by acute onset of symptoms after group A β-haemolytic streptococcal pharyngitis in prepubertal children. It has been postulated that the basal ganglia are involved in this process, a hypothesis that is supported by neuropsychological and neuroimaging evidence of basal ganglia dysfunction in both OCD and Sydenham's chorea.

Treatment of OCD can be difficult because of frequent relapses and incomplete response. Moderate or severe cases require cognitive behavioural therapy and treatment with drugs. Selective serotonin-reuptake inhibitors (SSRIs) are the first-line drug treatment for OCD. Major tranquillisers are effective drugs in schizophrenia but have no place in the treatment of OCD.

13.5   B: Tongue biting

Psychogenic non-epileptic seizures (pseudoseizures) have been linked to stress, anxiety and possible dissociative tendencies. Differentiating pseudoseizures from true epilepsy is difficult. This often results in a misdiagnosis and unnecessary and ineffective treatment. Certain behaviour, such as side-to-side turning of the head, asymmetric and large-amplitude shaking movements of the limbs, twitching of all four extremities without loss of consciousness, pelvic thrusting, and screaming or talking during the event, are more commonly associated with psychogenic rather than with epileptic seizures. Pseudo-status epilepticus may be more common than true status epilepticus. The patient may be incontinent but never exhibits tongue biting. Approximately 90% of patients are women and a 'role model' (a family history of epilepsy or experience of epilepsy in a paramedical occupation) is often present. However, the distinction is sometimes difficult to make on clinical grounds alone.

Prolonged EEG/video recording is the most sensitive tool for differentiating pseudoseizures from epilepsy, but is costly and therefore limited in availability. Measurement of serum prolactin levels may also help to discriminate between organic and psychogenic seizures, because most generalised seizures and many complex partial seizures are accompanied by rises in serum prolactin (during the immediate 30-minute postictal period) and psychogenic seizures are not.

13.6   A: Chromosomal analysis

This 18-year-old has fragile X syndrome and the most appropriate investigation is chromosomal analysis for a fragile X study. It is associated in a large proportion of gene carriers with a fragile site on the long arm of the X chromosome (Xq27.3). Fragile X syndrome occurs in 1 in 1000 male births; 1 in 3000 is the frequency in females, who are usually carriers but can express phenotypic features and mental retardation. Fragile X is the second most common known cause of mental retardation in males. The phenotype in males is large jaw (prognathism), large, low-set, floppy ears and large testes (macro-orchidism). They also have short stature, hyperflexible joints, attention deficit hyperactivity disorder (ADHD) and autistic-spectrum disorders.

13.7   C: Abnormal involuntary movements, typically choreoathetoid, which are usually complex, rapid and stereotyped

The most common presentation of tardive dyskinesia is chewing and pouting movements of the jaw and mouth (orobuccolingual dyskinesia). An early presentation is an inability to keep the tongue protruded from the mouth. Fixed contortions of the muscles of the head, neck and upper limbs are characteristic of acute dystonia, which can present as torticollis or as an oculogyric crisis, with involvement of limb muscles and upturning of the eyes. It occurs immediately or within a few days of treatment, unlike tardive dyskinesia, which usually occurs after at least 6 months of treatment. Muscular rigidity, tremor and bradykinesia are parkinsonian side-effects, which may occur acutely following antipsychotic drug administration and are commonest in older female patients. Tardive dyskinesia may be irreversible.

13.8   D: Delayed or absent grief

In 1998, Murray Parkes described abnormal grief as:

- unexpected grief, when the death occurs in a horrifying way and suddenly
- ambivalent grief, where the relationship with the deceased was disharmonious
- where the grief is chronic, though normal in nature; this kind of reaction occurs following a dependent relationship
- delayed or absent grief.

All the other answers are features of a normal grief reaction, as are sadness, weeping, poor sleep, reduced appetite and motor restlessness.

13.9   B: Delirium due to drug or alcohol withdrawal

The patient in the scenario has the hallmark features of delirium tremens. He has all the features of a delirium or acute organic brain syndrome. There is a fluctuating level of consciousness, global impairment of cognition (perceptual disturbance, disorientation and impaired attention), psychomotor abnormalities (hyper-alert), and an emotional disturbance. The specific diagnosis is suggested by his tremulousness, ataxia and the timing of the onset of the disturbance (approximately 48 hours after his last drink). It is also important to remember that between a third and a half of people with a major mental illness will misuse or be dependent on some form of drug, including alcohol.

Drug intoxication and related psychosis is also a possibility as drugs are available in hospital, but less likely given the continuous monitoring he received. A head injury is unlikely to present with such an evolution of symptoms, although this should be excluded in all patients with alcohol misuse. The neuroleptic malignant syndrome can present with a delirium and autonomic instability and rigidity. Non-organic causes of his symptoms are unlikely given the presence of delirium.

13.10   B: Paranoid schizophrenia

This patient describes several of the so-called 'first-rank symptoms' of schizophrenia:

1   **Auditory hallucinations:**

    • thoughts being spoken aloud
    • voices commenting on or discussing the individual in the third person (the voices keep saying things like, 'He is so stupid.').

2   **Thought disorder:**

    • thought withdrawal (eg 'The aliens are draining my thoughts with their rays.')
    • thought insertion (as with this patient)
    • thought broadcasting (eg 'The neighbours can hear what I'm thinking because of the special transmitter in my head.').

3   **Passivity experiences:**

    • 'made' actions, feelings or impulses (eg 'The aliens made me feel sad and cry by shining the rays of the machine on my head.').

4   **Delusional perception:**

    • the attaching of a delusional meaning to a normal precept (eg 'I saw the car and so I knew I was The Chosen One.').

These are not pathognomonic of schizophrenia (they can occur in mania and in epileptic psychosis) but when present over a long time make the diagnosis highly likely.

Bipolar affective disorder is suggested by the grandiose nature of his symptoms. However, the behaviour and affect is not that of a manic patient. Drug-induced psychoses can rarely give rise to elaborate symptoms (especially stimulants and hallucinogens) but the symptoms would not last for 9 months. Cotard's syndrome refers to nihilistic delusions, usually found in older depressed patients (eg 'All my insides have died and are disappearing,'). An organic schizophreniform disorder is a possibility and must be excluded, but an organic cause is rarely found for patients presenting with a classic symptom profile as described in this scenario.

13.11 D: Lewy bodies

The patient described has the characteristic features of Lewy body dementia. He has marked extrapyramidal signs, visual hallucinations and a variable symptom profile. He is also exquisitely sensitive to the anticholinergic side-effects of neuroleptics. Lewy bodies are eosinophilic inclusion bodies found within neurones, mainly in the limbic areas.

Neurofibrillary tangles and senile plaques are the characteristic histopathological findings in Alzheimer's disease. In Alzheimer's there is an early impairment of memory, which evolves into more general deficits in concentration and attention. Focal signs tend to appear late. Multiple infarct dementia classically runs a stepwise course, with an acute onset and patchy cognitive impairments. Personality is said to be preserved until relatively late in the course of the illness. Pick bodies are agyrophilic inclusions within neurones and are associated with frontotemporal dementias. Personality change is an early feature in this dementia, but tends to involve disinhibition, as might be expected with frontal pathology.

13.12 C: Akathisia

Movement disorders are a common and distressing side-effect of antipsychotic drugs. The most immediate complication is acute dystonia, which can arise hours to days after starting medication. This presents as fixed muscle postures with intense spasm. The classic presentation is of an oculogyric crisis, with the eyes deviated upwards and the head thrown backwards with a gaping mouth. Treatment is with an anticholinergic.

Extrapyramidal side-effects appear days to weeks after medication is started: there is rigidity, bradykinesia and increased tone, with a festinant gait and mask-like facies; patients are treated with an anticholinergic or by switching to one of the newer, atypical antipsychotics (such as risperidone, olanzapine or quetiapine), which are less likely to cause parkinsonism.

Akathisia is an intensely unpleasant combination of inner and outer restlessness. These patients are treated by reducing the dose of the antipsychotic, switching to a newer agent or with propranolol or a benzodiazepine; anticholinergics do not help.

Tardive dyskinesia presents with orofacial dyskinesia, with lip smacking, tongue protrusion and choreoathetoid movements of the head, neck and trunk. It appears months to years after starting medication. Treatment includes reducing all antipsychotic medication, if possible, or switching to clozapine (an atypical antipsychotic). It is often mistaken for a worsening of the underlying psychotic illness, which can lead to a disastrous increase in the dose of antipsychotic medication. Tardive dystonia presents with dystonic posturing and is characterised by its late onset, months to years after starting medication.

Chapter 14

RESPIRATORY MEDICINE

Answers

14.1 A: The PaO_2 at its best is not above 50 mmHg (7 kPa)

Persistent cyanosis without hypoxia (ie a normal PaO_2) suggests a diagnosis of methaemoglobinaemia, or sulph-haemoglobinaemia. In a cyanosed patient, the amount of reduced haemoglobin in the blood is at least 5 g/dl or more. The blue colour of the skin and mucous membrane is due to hypoxia and not to hypercapnia. Hypoxia should always be corrected with oxygen therapy.

14.2 C: Chest pain worse on deep breathing and a respiratory rate of 26 breaths/minute

The clinical features of pulmonary embolism (PE) can be diverse and confusing and range from no symptoms to sudden death. Sudden shortness of breath, pleuritic chest pain with haemoptysis and tachypnoea are the commonest features. However, a diagnosis that rests on clinical grounds alone is often incorrect. Several features, however, point away from the diagnosis of PE, including positive features of chest infection, such as swinging temperature (>39 °C) for more than a few days, associated with cough and purulent sputum. Recurrent chest pain in the same location is unusual in PE and it indicates an underlying diseased lung, such as bronchiectasis with recurrent chest infection. Haemoptysis in PE may be blood-tinged, blood-streaked or pure blood. It is rarely more than 5 ml or massive and seldom lasts for more than a few days. A normal chest X-ray is uncommon in acute PE but the usual findings, such as a small area of consolidation or a small pleural effusion, are not specific. Chest pain on lying flat is characteristic of pericarditis.

14.3   A: Asthma

The diffusion of carbon monoxide (CO) from the alveoli to the pulmonary blood is governed by the integrity of the alveolar membrane, the capillary blood volume, or both (the air–blood barrier). A reduction in the diffusion capacity of CO is encountered in conditions affecting the capillary bed size, such as pulmonary emboli and pulmonary vasculitis, or conditions that cause changes in the characteristics of the alveolar membrane, which include diseases in which some form of intra-alveolar filling process has occurred and the air–blood diffusion pathway is actually lengthened (pneumonia, pulmonary oedema, alveolar proteinosis). Similarly, the TLCO is reduced in patients with infiltrative disorders of the lung that affect both the capillary bed size and the alveolar membrane integrity, such as sarcoidosis, interstitial lung diseases, or collagen vascular diseases. Removal or destruction of lung tissue, as in surgical removal or emphysema, decreases both membrane and blood volume components and results in a low TLCO.

An increase in TLCO results occasionally from an increase in capillary blood volume secondary to haemodynamic changes in the pulmonary circulation: an increase in pulmonary arterial or left arterial pressures, as in congestive heart failure; or an increase in pulmonary blood flow, as in atrial septal defect. The TLCO is sometimes increased in patients with bronchial asthma during an attack, but the cause of this change is not known. Alveolar haemorrhage from any cause can result in a false increase of TLCO despite the presence of an underlying diffusion defect.

14.4   D: Six weeks of postpartum warfarin therapy is recommended after completion of anticoagulation during the pregnancy

Compression of the common iliac vein by the gravid uterus is responsible for the venous stasis in the lower limbs during pregnancy. The majority of deep venous thromboses (DVTs) occurring during pregnancy are found in the left leg, most probably because of compression of the left iliac vein by the crossing right iliac artery at its origin from the aorta. The vast majority of DVTs in pregnancy are iliofemoral and will therefore require treatment. Isolated below-knee DVT is uncommon.

Any woman with signs and symptoms suggestive of venous thromboembolism should have objective testing performed expeditiously to avoid the risks, inconvenience and costs of inappropriate anticoagulation. Following delivery, treatment should continue for at least 6–12 weeks. Warfarin can be used following delivery. Systematic reviews have concluded that LMW heparin is a safe alternative to unfractionated heparin for anticoagulation during pregnancy. Furthermore, long-term use of LMW heparins may be associated with a lower risk of osteoporosis and bone fractures than unfractionated heparin.

14.5   C: Auscultation of the lungs usually reveals no abnormality

Pneumocystis carinii pneumonia (PCP) is a pulmonary disease characterised by dyspnoea, tachypnoea and hypoxaemia that occurs in patients deficient in immunoglobulins G and M, and in patients deficient in cell-mediated immunity. The vast majority of adult patients have AIDS, but it can also occur in patients who have received chemotherapy for haematological malignancy or post-organ transplant. It can also occur in malnourished or premature infants. On examination, patients usually show signs of respiratory distress (tachypnoea, dyspnoea). Auscultation of the lungs usually reveals no abnormalities. The trophozoite does not enter the blood; the organism is identified in pulmonary secretions obtained by bronchoalveolar lavage or lung biopsy and stained by methenamine silver or Giemsa stain. Pentamidine isetionate or co-trimoxazole is the recommended treatment (metronidazole is not effective in the treatment of PCP).

14.6   B: Pancreatic insufficiency is almost always identified in adult patients

Cystic fibrosis is an autosomal recessive disease which affects both eccrine and exocrine gland function and is characterised by elevated levels of sodium and chloride in the sweat. It is caused by abnormally viscid secretions from mucous glands that lead to chronic pulmonary disease and pancreatic insufficiency, which will be evident in more than 95% of adult patients. The carrier rate is 5% in the Caucasian population; heterozygotes are clinically normal. Recurrent chest infections are usually caused by

Pseudomonas aeruginosa and *Staphylococcus aureus.*
Pseudomonas cepacia is found in 5–10% of cases.

14.7 B: Complete remission without any specific treatment

Acute sarcoidosis comprises the complex of erythema nodosum
and X-ray findings of bilateral hilar adenopathy, often
accompanied by joint symptoms, including arthritis at the ankles,
knees, wrists or elbows. Spontaneous remission occurs in nearly
two-thirds of patients with acute sarcoidosis, while 10–30%
develop a chronic form of the disease. Remission often occurs
within the first 6 months after diagnosis. Non-steroidal anti-
inflammatory drugs (NSAIDs) are very useful for controlling
musculoskeletal symptoms.

14.8 B: It may be associated with hyponatraemia

Small-cell (oat-cell) bronchial carcinoma is frequently associated
with ectopic hormone production: the syndrome of inappropriate
antidiuretic hormone secretion (SIADH) causes hyponatraemia.
By the time the diagnosis has been made, the tumour is usually
disseminated, so that surgery is seldom considered. Unlike
mesothelioma, a history of asbestos exposure is seldom obtained.
The prognosis is very poor and survival beyond 2 years is
exceptional.

14.9 D: Exacerbations are related to cooling of the airway

The mechanism involves inhalation of cold air, cooling of the
airway and an increase in the osmolarity of the lining fluid, which
causes release of mediators and stimulates vagal efferent
pathways. It is more common in children than in adults. Sodium
cromoglicate or β-agonists may blunt or prevent symptoms when
given by inhalation before exercise; inhaled steroids are
ineffective. Inhaled pollens are antigens that can induce
bronchospasm in any type of asthma and this is not more common
in exercise-induced asthma.

14.10 B: Löeffler's syndrome

Eosinophilic lung diseases are a heterogeneous group of disorders which are characterised by the presence of pulmonary symptoms or an abnormal chest X-ray accompanied by an inflammatory cell infiltrate in the airways and/or lung parenchyma, which contains a large number of eosinophils. Many of these disorders are associated with peripheral eosinophilia. The following are just a few examples:

- drugs and toxins, eg nitrofurantoin, L-tryptophan, sulphonamides
- helminthic infections, eg Löeffler's syndrome, larva migrans
- acute and chronic eosinophilic pneumonia (primary)
- Churg–Strauss syndrome
- allergic bronchopulmonary aspergillosis
- hypereosinophilic syndrome.

14.11 D: A positive tuberculin test in chronic cases is suggestive of concomitant tuberculosis

Sarcoidosis is a systemic disorder of unknown cause that is characterised by its pathological hallmark, the non-caseating granuloma, which primarily affects the respiratory tract, skin, eyes, heart, kidneys and liver. Pleural disease is relatively uncommon, with effusions occurring in fewer than 5% of patients. Finger clubbing is not a recognised feature of sarcoidosis. Although liver biopsy reveals granulomatous involvement in 40–70% of patients, clinically significant hepatic disease is rare. A tuberculin test is usually negative in chronic sarcoidosis, although most sarcoidosis patients who develop tuberculosis become tuberculin-positive. Hypercalcaemia, a potentially important complication of sarcoidosis, occurs in fewer than 10% of patients and is thought to be due to elevated levels of 1,25-dihydroxy-vitamin D (calcitriol), which is produced by macrophages in the granulomas. High-dose glucocorticoids are very helpful in the treatment of hypercalcaemia due to vitamin D intoxication, granulomatous diseases such as sarcoidosis and in haematological malignancies known to be, or likely to be, glucocorticoid-responsive.

14.12 C: The scan findings are more informative if the chest X-ray is normal

Ventilation-perfusion imaging is most valuable in patients

suspected of having pulmonary embolism who have a normal chest X-ray. Two or more segmental perfusion defects, which are associated with normal regional ventilation (ie mismatched) have a high probability of representing pulmonary embolism, whereas perfusion defects that are associated with a ventilatory abnormality of comparable size (ie matched) are more likely to reflect regional hypoperfusion secondary to airway disease. Mismatch in perfusion and ventilation can also be caused by old pulmonary embolism, vasculitis, previous irradiation therapy, arteriovenous malformation, congenital pulmonary artery lesions and compression or invasion of pulmonary vessels by hilar or mediastinal masses. The sensitivity of perfusion imaging is high, so a normal perfusion study effectively excludes pulmonary embolism.

14.13 C: Persistent hypoxaemia, PaO_2 <7.3 kPa

The role of long-term oxygen therapy for hypoxaemia in patients with chronic obstructive pulmonary disease (COPD) is well established and clinical trials conducted in the 1980s have proved its efficacy in this condition. Oxygen therapy has been shown to increase the life expectancy of patients with moderate to severe hypoxaemia.

UK criteria for long-term oxygen (oxygen therapy for between 15 and 24 hours a day):

- PaO_2 <7.3 kPa
- $PaCO_2$ >6 kPa
- FEV_1 <1.5 litres
- FVC <2.0 litres.

Measurements should be stable over 3 weeks and taken when the patient is receiving optimal medical treatment.

14.14 A: *Streptococcus pneumoniae*

Community-acquired pneumonia is contracted in the community rather than in hospital. In the northern hemisphere, community-acquired pneumonia affects approximately 12 per 1000 people per year, particularly during winter and at the extremes of age (the incidence is 30–50/1000/year in infants under 12 months; and

50/1000/year in 71–85-year-olds). Over a hundred micro-
organisms have been implicated, but most cases are caused by
Streptococcus pneumoniae. Smoking is probably an important
risk factor.

14.15   A: In diaphragmatic paralysis it occurs immediately after lying down

Dyspnoea in a patient with diaphragmatic paralysis occurs
immediately following lying down. This happens because the
abdominal contents displace the flaccid diaphragm upwards into
the thorax. The onset of shortness of breath 2–3 hours after the
onset of sleep is characteristic of paroxysmal nocturnal dyspnoea
resulting from increased left atrial pressure. In dyspnoea from
almost any organic cause, it is unlikely that the symptoms will
improve or remain unchanged during exercise, but dyspnoea
occurring 10 minutes after the cessation of exercise is
characteristic of exercise-induced bronchospasm. The offending
antigen in hypersensitivity pneumonitis induces an Arthus-like
reaction that requires 6–8 hours to develop after the exposure and
dyspnoea may not occur until late afternoon – typically, the
symptoms improve at the weekend, as there is no further exposure
to the antigen.

14.16   B: Immotile cilia syndrome (Kartagener's syndrome)

This patient has familial bronchiectasis. Bronchiectasis may be
caused by congenital diseases that cause structural damage in the
lung or impair immunity. Other causes include IgM deficiency,
α_1-antitrypsin deficiency and cystic fibrosis.

14.17   E: Low sensitivity for detecting pulmonary emboli in subsegmental pulmonary arteries

The development of fast scanning techniques with helical (spiral)
computed tomography (CT) scanners has facilitated the use of this
tool in the diagnosis of acute and chronic pulmonary embolism.
Spiral CT scanning allows imaging of the entire chest with
intravenous contrast enhancement during a single breath-hold.
The majority of studies performed to date have shown CT
angiography to be an accurate, non-invasive tool in the diagnosis

of pulmonary embolism at the main, lobar and segmental pulmonary artery levels. However, CT angiography is less accurate in imaging peripheral emboli in the subsegmental arteries. The sensitivity and specificity is generally regarded as being comparable to that of standard pulmonary angiography. Technical factors may account for approximately 5–10% of CT angiograms being non-diagnostic, but this figure is comparable to that of standard pulmonary angiography.

14.18 D: Cephalosporin + aminoglycoside

This patient has a hospital-acquired pneumonia, the third most common hospital-acquired infection after urinary tract infections and wound infections. Because they occur in hospital, the pathogens involved are very different from those that cause community-acquired pneumonia. Gram-negative organisms are far more common because:

- colonisation of the oropharynx by Gram-negative bacilli is very common in hospitalised patients, who have often been on broad-spectrum antibiotics already
- there is an increased risk of micro-aspiration of nasopharyngeal secretions
- patients in hospital often have depressed immune systems.

Antibiotics that will cover such organisms should therefore be started, usually as a combination therapy: a third-generation cephalosporin with an aminoglycoside is the present British Thoracic Society (BTS) recommendation.

14.19 C: Chest X-ray

Chronic cough is defined as cough that persists for more than 8 weeks. Chronic cough can have many causes. In most cases, an underlying cause can be identified by taking a thorough history and performing a detailed physical examination. In immunocompetent adults who are not taking an angiotensin-converting enzyme (ACE) inhibitor, a chest X-ray should be the first test obtained to rule out malignancy and other serious conditions. If the chest X-ray is essentially normal, one has to think of the 'pathogenic triad of chronic cough', which comprises postnasal drip syndrome, asthma and gastro-oesophageal reflux disease (GORD). This disease triad accounts for nearly all cases of chronic cough in non-smokers who have essentially normal chest X-rays and who are not taking an ACE inhibitor. Radiography of the sinuses may be useful for confirming the diagnosis of sinusitis as the cause of postnasal drip syndrome. Postnasal drip syndrome which is not caused by sinusitis consistently responds to the combination of a decongestant and a first-generation H_1-receptor antagonist antihistamine.

After postnasal drip syndrome, asthma is the next most common cause of chronic cough in immunocompetent adults. Pulmonary function tests with a methacholine challenge test are appropriate for patients with suspected asthma. A methacholine challenge test is recommended because a negative result effectively rules out asthma. The most sensitive and specific test for GORD is 24-hour oesophageal pH monitoring. Because of the inconvenience of this test, however, it is not recommended in the routine evaluation of GORD. An alternative approach is the empiric use of antireflux medications such as proton pump inhibitors or H_2-receptor antagonist antihistamines. If the cause of chronic cough remains unclear, high-resolution CT scanning of the chest and bronchoscopy may be indicated.

14.20 B: Mandibular advancement splinting

Obstructive sleep apnoea is caused by loss of upper airway/pharyngeal muscle tone during rapid eye movement (REM) sleep, which leads to airway obstruction and consequent apnoeic episodes. It affects 1–2% of middle-aged men. Good first-line treatments in most patients are simple measures, such as weight loss and alcohol avoidance. Surgery is really a last-ditch attempt to solve the problem. Many trials have looked at the effectiveness of both mandibular advancement splints (a tailor-made mouthpiece which helps to keep the jaw forward and aids upper airway muscle tone when asleep) and continuous positive airway pressure (CPAP) ventilation. Both seem to be effective and are comparable in efficacy. Long-term oxygen therapy is really only an adjunct treatment for patients who have other coexistent lung pathologies.

Chapter 15

RHEUMATOLOGY AND IMMUNOLOGY

Answers

15.1 C: Scleritis

Episcleritis is the most common cause of a painless red eye in rheumatoid arthritis. It is encountered in 10–20% of cases. The pupils and retina are typically normal. It does not warrant specific treatment as such. It usually improves with better control of the disease. Scleritis is usually painful and more serious. It usually requires topical or systemic treatment. Fortunately, it is less common than episcleritis. Iritis is associated with red, painful, congested eyes and small pupils. The retina is usually abnormal in macular degeneration and posterior uveitis.

15.2 B: Give 60 mg of prednisolone orally

This patient's symptoms are typical of temporal arteritis. Oral steroids should be started immediately to control the disease and prevent sudden loss of vision, which is a recognised complication of untreated disease.

15.3 B: It provides immunity against tuberculosis for 5–10 years

The vaccine contains live attenuated *Mycobacterium bovis*. Immunity usually lasts for 5–10 years. The side-effects of the vaccine include infection at the injection site and regional lymphadenopathy. Most developing countries give the vaccine to all newborn babies unless there is a contraindication. The tuberculin test becomes positive after vaccination.

15.4   D: C1 esterase inhibitor level

Angio-oedema, characterised by non-pitting, erythematous swelling of soft tissues, can be hereditary or acquired. Hereditary angio-oedema is characterised by recurrent self-limited attacks involving the skin, subcutaneous tissue, upper respiratory tract, or gastrointestinal tract. Attacks may last from several hours to 2–3 days. Gastrointestinal or upper respiratory tract attacks may be precipitated by local trauma (eg dental procedures, tonsillectomy).

Hereditary angio-oedema is an autosomal dominant disease caused by mutations in the C1 esterase inhibitor gene. The defective gene does not produce sufficient levels of C1 esterase inhibitor in plasma, which leads to auto-activation of C1 and consumption of C2 and C4. The disorder is further classified into type I (lower production of C1 esterase inhibitor proteins) and type II (functional defect of C1 esterase inhibitor with normal plasma levels), detectable by an immune assay. Between attacks, low levels of C4 are noted. Acquired angio-oedema may be a manifestation of urticaria; it has recently been described with drugs such as angiotensin-converting enzyme (ACE) inhibitors.

15.5   D: Monoclonal gammopathy of undetermined significance (MGUS)

The incidence of monoclonal gammopathy of undetermined significance (MGUS) increases with age, from 1% at the age of 25 years to 4% in the over-70s. Many cases are seemingly benign. However, up to 25% progress to a B-cell malignancy or myeloma, which may not become clinically apparent for more than 20 years. The course is impossible to predict. Investigations usually show: low M-protein levels in serum (< 3 g/dl) or urine (< 300 mg/24 hours), which are stable over time; normal levels of other serum immunoglobulins; no lytic bone lesions; no Bence Jones proteinuria; and only mild plasmacytosis in the bone marrow. No treatment is recommended. Patients should be observed for clinical and immunochemical changes every 4–6 months.

The small M band, absent lytic lesions and negative Bence Jones proteinuria would probably exclude multiple myeloma as a possible diagnosis in a fit elderly man. The diagnosis of

Waldenström's macroglobulinaemia is established by demonstrating a typical M spike on serum protein electrophoresis that proves to be IgM on immunoelectrophoresis or immunofixation. Similar blood abnormalities are also associated with rheumatoid arthritis and carcinoma of the prostate. In these circumstances, serum M components may represent unusual antibody responses to protracted antigenic stimuli. However, the clinical features in this case are not suggestive of any of these conditions.

15.6   A: The erythrocyte sedimentation rate (ESR) is elevated in hypoalbuminaemia

Fibrinogen, an acute-phase protein, contributes > 90% of the plasma viscosity due to its high molecular weight and marked asymmetry. During an acute pathological process, the rise in plasma viscosity is primarily due to an increase in plasma fibrinogen levels. In chronic organic disease, the increase in plasma viscosity is caused by persistent elevation of fibrinogen and serum globulins, with an associated fall in albumin levels in plasma. The plasma viscosity is more specific and more sensitive than the ESR. C-reactive protein (CRP) is an acute-phase reactant protein and it is produced in the liver. Its levels are typically normal in active systemic lupus erythematosus and in primary Sjögren's syndrome.

15.7   D: Wegener's granulomatosis

Wegener's granulomatosis is a primary small-vessel vasculitis which involves the kidneys and causes glomerulonephritis with crescent formation. It is distinguished from other causes of glomerulonephritis by the absence of immune deposits on immunohistochemical analysis.

15.8   B: The liver clears IgM-sensitised erythrocytes

Class II MHC antigens are crucial to antigen recognition and presentation and are found on B lymphocytes, monocyte-macrophages and activated T lymphocytes. IgG-sensitised erythrocytes are cleared by the spleen while IgM-sensitised erythrocytes are cleared by the liver. C5a causes the release of non-IgE-dependent mediators from mast cells, to increase vascular permeability and to induce smooth-muscle contraction. C3b, not C5a, is the complement fragment that activates the alternative pathway. Paroxysmal nocturnal haemoglobinuria is a condition in which there is a clonal abnormality in erythrocytes, which make them more susceptible to complement-mediated lytic attack, leading to intravascular haemolysis.

15.9   E: Hepatitis C infection

The term 'cryoglobulinaemia' refers to the presence in the serum of one (monoclonal cryoimmunoglobulinaemia) or more immunoglobulins (mixed cryoglobulinaemia), which precipitate at temperatures below 37 °C and re-dissolve on rewarming. Three different types of cryoglobulins have been described. The cryoglobulins in type II essential mixed cryoglobulinaemia (EMC) contain both a polyclonal IgG and a monoclonal IgM rheumatoid factor directed against the IgG. Palpable purpura occurs in the great majority of patients with mixed essential cryoglobulinaemia and this is an important clue to the diagnosis. Glomerulonephritis occurs in a substantial minority and is a major cause of death. Cold intolerance is more likely to be a feature of type I cryoglobulinaemia than of EMC. Rheumatoid factor is positive and complement levels are usually depressed in EMC. Although infections with Epstein–Barr virus and hepatitis B virus have been implicated in some cases, it now seems clear that most cases are due to chronic infection with hepatitis C virus.

Osteolytic lesions and Bence Jones proteins are features of multiple myeloma. Cold agglutinins are not a feature of cryoglobulinaemia. Cold agglutinins or cold autoantibodies occur naturally in nearly everyone. These natural cold autoantibodies occur at low titres (less than 1 in 64, measured at 4 °C) and have no activity at higher temperatures. Pathological cold agglutinins occur at titres of over 1 in 1000 and react at 28–31 °C. Cold agglutinins react with polysaccharide antigens of the ABO system present on the red blood cells of all humans. Cold agglutinins attach to the red blood cells in the cooler peripheral circulation and dissociate from the red blood cells as the blood returns to the warmer central circulation. Cold agglutinins cause autoimmune haemolytic anaemia.

15.10 E: The fingers are symmetrically involved during an attack

	Primary Raynaud's phenomenon	Secondary Raynaud's phenomenon
Average age, years	15	> 40
Gender	Female	Male
Tissue damage	Absent	Digital ulcers, gangrene
Symmetry	Symmetrical	Asymmetrical
Capillaroscopy	Negative	Positive
Autoantibodies	Negative	Positive
Associated diseases	None	Scleroderma, systemic lupus erythematosus, other connective tissue diseases

15.11 D: Peripheral asymmetrical oligoarthropathy

Peripheral oligoarthropathy is the most common presentation of psoriatic arthropathy and accounts for 35–40% of all cases. It usually presents with an asymmetrical pattern of large- and small-joint involvement. Symmetrical polyarthropathy resembling rheumatoid arthritis may occur in 20–30% of patients. Psoriatic spondylitis accounts for approximately 20% of cases. Synovitis of the DIP joints of the hands, often in the joints adjacent to affected nails, is almost pathognomonic of psoriatic arthropathy but occurs in less than 10% of all cases. Arthritis mutilans is uncommon (< 5%).

15.12 B: Positive anticardiolipin antibodies

Antiphospholipid syndrome is characterised by thrombosis of arteries and veins, recurrent abortions and thrombocytopenia. It was first described in systemic lupus erythematosus (SLE), but has since been described in a wide range of autoimmune diseases, associated with a variety of autoimmune autoantibodies. It may also present in isolation in the primary antiphospholipid syndrome. Antiphospholipid antibodies are immunoglobulins of the IgG and IgM classes, which are directed against a negatively charged phospholipid molecule. The presence of antiphospholipid antibodies may be suggested by the presence of lupus anticoagulant, a prolonged activated partial thromboplastin time, a false-positive VDRL, or by anticardiolipin antibodies (measured by radioimmunoassay or enzyme-linked immunosorbent assay). Although there is an increased risk of atherosclerosis and ischaemic heart disease in patients with SLE and antiphospholipid syndrome, elevated low density lipoproteins is not a feature of the primary condition. Complement levels are generally normal in this disorder.

15.13 C: Alveolar-cell carcinoma of the lung is a recognised complication

The pulmonary hypertension is caused by an avascular obliterative process, which is the hallmark of systemic sclerosis. Some patients have sclerodermal visceral disease without cutaneous involvement (systemic sclerosis sine scleroderma). Trigeminal neuralgia and alveolar-cell carcinoma are rare but recognised complications. The skin changes extend proximal to the MCP joints, a feature that helps to differentiate it from limited cutaneous sclerosis (CREST syndrome). In uncomplicated cases the ESR is typically within normal limits. The ESR is a poor indicator of disease activity in systemic sclerosis.

15.14 B: Tenosynovitis

In the early stages of the disease there is polyarthritis affecting the wrist and hand joints, but this is soon replaced by a monoarthritis once the disease is established. Synovial smear and culture tests are often negative. The synovial effusion often contains more than 100 000 leucocytes/mm³. In gonococcal arthritis there is a high frequency of associated tenosynovitis and skin rash (vesiculopostural with an erythematous base) – both are characteristic. Resistance to penicillin is uncommon. The risk of dissemination is greater in females and is particularly high during menstruation, pregnancy, the postpartum period, and in individuals with a genetic deficiency in the terminal components of the serum complement system (C5, C6, C7 or C8). Episcleritis is a feature of seropositive inflammatory arthropathies such as rheumatoid arthritis.

15.15 B: Antiribonucleoprotein antibody (anti-RNP)

The patient's clinical features are highly suggestive of mixed connective tissue disease (MCTD). This diagnosis has been applied to a particular subset of patients with overlapping clinical features of lupus, scleroderma and myositis. An immune response to U1-RNP is the additional defining serological feature of MCTD. Homogeneous antinuclear antibodies are more common in patients with systemic lupus erythematosus.

15.16 C: Serum ferritin

This patient has pseudogout. The plain X-ray of the knee will show linear calcification of the knee cartilage (chondrocalcinosis). This is due to calcium pyrophosphate dihydrate (CPPD) crystal deposition. In a young patient, chondrocalcinosis may be an important clue to a number of systemic diseases, including:

- hyperparathyroidism
- haemochromatosis
- hypothyroidism
- ochronosis
- hypophosphatasia
- hypomagnesaemia
- acromegaly
- Wilson's disease.

Chondrocalcinosis can also complicate gout and rheumatoid arthritis. Addison's disease and Cushing's syndrome are not associated with an increased incidence of crystal-induced synovitis.

15.17 A: Spinal cord compression due to cervical myelopathy from atlanto-axial subluxation

This patient exhibits upper motor neurone signs affecting the upper and lower limbs. The most probable diagnosis is cervical myelopathy secondary to rheumatoid arthritis. The hallmark symptoms of cervical myelopathy are weakness or stiffness in the legs and weakness or clumsiness of the hands. Loss of sphincter control or frank incontinence is rare; however, some patients may complain of slight hesitancy. A characteristic physical finding in cervical myelopathy is hyper-reflexia; there may also be ankle clonus and a positive Babinski sign. Magnetic resonance imaging

(MRI) of the cervical spine is the investigation of choice during the initial screening of patients with suspected cervical myelopathy.

Subcutaneous rheumatoid nodules occur in 20–25% of patients. These are usually observed in areas subject to pressure, such as the elbows, the occiput or the sacrum. The central nervous system is usually spared. In myasthenia gravis and disuse muscle atrophy, the Babinski sign is negative.

15.18 C: Ankylosing spondylitis

The character of the back pain suggests inflammatory disease. The pain has persisted for over 3 months. He has noticed increasing back stiffness in the morning that improves during the day; the pain is probably so severe at night that it prompts him to get up and move about to reduce the symptoms. These features suggest inflammatory pain, most probably due to ankylosing spondylitis. Patients with ankylosing spondylitis generally present with back pain that is worse after rest and improves with exercise. The typical patient is a man under 40, and the onset is typically insidious.

Sciatica is the symptomatic hallmark of clinically significant disc herniation. It presents as sharp or burning pain which radiates down the posterior or lateral aspect of the leg to the ankle or foot (depending on the specific nerve root involved). The pain may be worsened by cough, the Valsalva manoeuvre, or by sneezing and is often accompanied by paraesthesiae and numbness. Around 90% of mechanically-caused back pain lasts less than 8 weeks. Spinal canal stenosis occurs in young people who have a congenitally narrowed lumbar spinal canal and also in elderly people with osteoarthritic spurring, chronic disc degeneration, and facet-joint arthritis. The characteristic complaint is pain in the lower back and gluteal region that is exacerbated by standing, walking, or other activities that cause spinal extension. Other characteristics are relief by rest, especially by sitting or lying down, and flexing of the spine and hips. Because symptoms are often worsened by walking and they can mimic vascular insufficiency, this condition is sometimes referred to as 'pseudoclaudication'.

Back pain due to osteomyelitis is usually dull, and is often accompanied by low-grade fever and spasm over the paraspinous muscles. Tenderness to percussion over the involved vertebrae is common, but fever is absent in up to 50% of cases. Malignant vertebral deposits often present with severe, deep-seated pain that is worse at night and provoked by spine movement. In patients with malignant or infectious backache, the disease process is rapidly progressive and serious compression fractures or an epidural abscess may ensue. The fact that this patient remained stable 6 months after presentation makes such a diagnosis unlikely.

	Mechanical back pain	Inflammatory back pain
Onset	Acute	Insidious
Morning stiffness	+++	–
Effect of exercise	Worse	Better
Radiation	L5/S1 dermatomes	Diffuse
Neurological signs	Present	Absent

15.19 A: Lymphoma

The presence of objective evidence of dry mouth and/or dry eyes in a patient presenting with sicca symptoms and a positive anti-Ro antibody test is highly suggestive of Sjögren's syndrome. This is a chronic inflammatory disorder characterised primarily by diminished lacrimal and salivary gland secretions, resulting in symptoms of dry eyes and dry mouth. Sjögren's syndrome is characterised by polyclonal B-cell activation and lymphocytic infiltration of the exocrine glands. The risk of non-Hodgkin's lymphoma is said to be 44 times higher than in the normal population, with an individual risk of approximately 4–10%.

Parotid enlargement is due to lymphatic cell infiltration occurring as a manifestation of chronic inflammation and is not due to adenoma. Although there is an increased incidence of primary biliary cirrhosis and of chronic active hepatitis in patients with Sjögren's syndrome, there is no reported increase in the incidence of hepatoma. Renal tubular acidosis is a recognised complication of Sjögren's syndrome but there is no increase in the incidence of renal cell carcinoma.

15.20 C: Polyarteritis nodosa

This patient presents with generalised features, abdominal pain, hypertension and mononeuritis. The raised erythrocyte sedimentation rate and polymorphonuclear leucocytosis consolidate the possibility of a vasculitis, namely polyarteritis nodosa. The abdominal pain is highly suggestive of mesenteric ischaemia. Mononeuritis multiplex develops because of involvement of the vasa vasorum; it is reflected in this patient in his sudden loss of dorsiflexion of his left great toe. Wegener's granulomatosis and Churg–Strauss syndrome are commonly associated with pulmonary manifestations, which are absent in this case (the chest X-ray was normal). Systemic lupus erythematosus is more common in young women. Polymyalgia rheumatica presents with pain and stiffness in the shoulder and pelvic girdles, but hypertension and mononeuritis are not recognised features.

15.21 B: Fibromyalgia syndrome

Fibromyalgia syndrome (FMS) is a commonly encountered syndrome characterised by diffuse, persistent musculoskeletal pain, stiffness, tenderness, sleep disturbance and easy fatiguability. It predominantly affects women in the 30–60-year age range. The American College of Rheumatology (ACR) 1990 criteria for the classification of FMS include:

1   History of widespread pain which has been present for at least 3 months.

2   Pain must be present in at least 11 of the following 18 tender point sites on digital palpation: occiput (2), low cervical (2), trapezius (2), supraspinatus (2), second rib (2), lateral epicondyle (2), gluteal (2), greater trochanter (2), knee (2).

On physical examination, patients with primary FMS usually appear well, with no obvious systemic illness or articular abnormalities. Tenderness is the feature that most readily allows separation of FMS from other disorders that produce widespread pain or fatigue, such as chronic fatigue syndrome. Laboratory and radiological investigations in FMS are largely unrevealing and are primarily useful in searching for the presence of concomitant disorders. Even among normal blood donors, the incidence of a positive ANA is approximately 5% when the screening is done with a serum dilution of 1 in 40. The titre of the ANA test is usually over 1 in 160 in the systemic connective tissue diseases. Certain rheumatic and non-rheumatic diseases can also mimic FMS, with similar pain and fatigue, and must be considered and treated, even when FMS has been positively identified (examples include depression and hypothyroidism).

15.22 A: Diabetes mellitus is the most common cause

The mechanism that leads to the development of neuropathic joints is impairment of proprioceptive and pain sensations, which deprives the affected joint of the normal protective reactions that ordinarily modulate the forces of weight-bearing and motion. It can be a complication of a variety of neurological disorders; diabetic neuropathy is the most common. Poliomyelitis is an acute viral illness that selectively destroys the motor neurones. It does not cause loss of sensation or proprioception and so is not a cause of neuropathic joints.

Affected joints are grossly deformed, with significant swelling, reflecting a severe degree of destruction and disorganisation. The basic neurological lesion determines the distribution of the affected joints: in diabetic neuropathy, the changes are limited to the distal lower extremities and in syringomyelia the shoulder and elbows are most commonly affected. Total joint replacement has been attempted, but success has been limited and most consider this approach contraindicated.

15.23 D: Microscopic polyangiitis

ANCA can be detected in almost all patients with Wegener's granulomatosis. These antibodies are also found in 90% of cases of two related disorders with identical renal histological findings to Wegener's granulomatosis: microscopic polyangiitis, in which there are systemic symptoms that are not classic for Wegener's granulomatosis, and idiopathic necrotising glomerulonephritis. Approximately 70% of patients with Churg–Strauss syndrome (allergic angiitis and granulomatosis) are also ANCA-positive. In contrast, ANCA are much less common in classic polyarteritis nodosa, in which small- and medium-sized arteries are affected, occurring in approximately 20% of cases. Microscopic polyangiitis is associated with pANCA while Wegener's granulomatosis is associated with cANCA (cytoplasmic-staining ANCA). Takayasu's disease and giant-cell arteritis are large-vessel vasculitides and are rarely associated with glomerulonephritis. Systemic lupus erythematosus and Goodpasture's syndrome are associated with glomerulonephritis but not with high levels of ANCA.

15.24 D: Eclampsia of pregnancy

Pre-eclampsia and eclampsia are characteristically associated with low uric acid levels. The concentration of urate in plasma is determined by the balance between absorption and production of purines on the one hand and destruction and excretion on the other. There are very few causes of a low urate level (which, in itself, causes no ill effects).

In contrast, high uric acid levels are associated with significant morbidity. Causes of an increased uric acid level include:

- increased purine biosynthesis
- Lesch–Nyhan syndrome
- glucose-6-phosphatase deficiency (von Gierke's disease)
- increased nucleic acid turnover
- haemolysis, polycythaemia rubra vera
- reduced renal clearance
- chronic renal failure, lead poisoning, diuretics.

15.25 B: Polymyositis

Symmetrical proximal muscle weakness resulting from muscle inflammation is seen in polymyositis. Dysphagia, dysphonia and respiratory weakness may develop. Diagnosis is by measurement of creatine kinase, electromyography (EMG) and muscle biopsy.

Polymyalgia rheumatica is common in older women and presents as aching and morning stiffness in the proximal muscles. There is no muscle tenderness and the reflexes are normal. Hypocalcaemia presents with tetany, depression, carpopedal spasm and neuromuscular excitability (Chvostek's sign). Painful arc syndrome may be due to supraspinatus tendonitis, subacromial bursitis or calcification of the rotator cuff. This is usually unilateral. In frozen shoulder, there is marked reduction of passive and active movement. Abduction to even 90° is impossible, but muscle wasting, tenderness and reduced tendon reflexes are not seen.

Chapter 16

STATISTICS

Answers

16.1   C: The mean is higher than the median in a positively skewed distribution

The mean is a good measure of central tendency for roughly symmetric distributions but can be misleading in skewed distributions because it can be greatly influenced by extreme scores. Other statistics, such as the median, may therefore be more informative for distributions such as reaction times or family income that are frequently very skewed. For normal distributions, the mean is the most efficient (and therefore the least subject to sample fluctuations) of all measures of central tendency.

The median is the middle of a distribution (half the scores are above the median and half are below the median). The median is less sensitive to extreme scores than the mean and this makes it a better measure than the mean for highly skewed distributions: the median income is usually more informative than the mean income, for example. When there is an odd number of numbers, the median is simply the middle number when the numbers are arranged in order of magnitude: for example, the median of 2, 4, and 7 is 4. When there is an even number of numbers, the median is the mean of the two middle numbers: for example, the median of the numbers 2, 4, 7, and 12 is $(4 + 7) \div 2 = 5.5$.

The mean, median and mode are equal in symmetric distributions. The mean is higher than the median in positively skewed distributions and lower than the median in negatively skewed distributions.

The mode is the most frequently occurring score in a distribution. The advantage of the mode as a measure of central tendency is that its meaning is obvious. Furthermore, it is the only measure of central tendency that can be used with nominal data. The mode is greatly subject to sample fluctuations, however, and is therefore not recommended to be used as the only measure of central tendency. A further disadvantage of the mode is that many distributions have more than one mode. These distributions are known as 'multimodal'.

16.2   C: For every five people who smoke, one has the disease

The odds in a given group (in this case, smokers) are defined as the number with the disease/number without the disease. Because the odds here are 1/4 (ie for every one smoker with the disease, four do not have the disease), out of every five people who smoke, one will have the disease.

16.3   C: Nothing conclusive can be claimed; a larger study is required

Because 0/31 babies had serious side-effects, this does not mean that no infants ever will, so the drug has not been shown to be safe. If 3% of infants were to have serious side-effects from taking the drug, then we would only expect to have one out of a sample of 30 babies affected and it would not be that surprising if none were affected. A larger study is required to try and obtain a more precise estimate of the percentage of babies who will suffer from serious side-effects.

16.4   C: Mann–Whitney *U*-test

Although the best answer to this question is C, all the other answers have some virtue. Pain is measured here using an 'ordinal categorical' scale. Frequently, such scales are considered to be continuous (more correctly, pseudo-continuous) and the literature contains many instances of this practice. If this approximation is made, then options B and E are both appropriate tests – one-way analysis of variance is identical mathematically to an unpaired Student's *t*-test when only two groups are being compared. However, approximating to a continuous scale is problematic here: there are only four points on the scale; each point is given a specific definition; and the distances between the points are unlikely to be equal (moving from 'mild to 'moderate' will not

necessarily be the same as moving from 'moderate' to 'severe').
Strictly, both tests also require the data to follow a normal
(Gaussian) distribution – this is unlikely with a short ordinal scale.
Options B and E are thus the least desirable.

Options A and D are also effectively the same test. Both take the
extreme opposite view to that adopted above and treat the pain
scale as being wholly categorical (ie 'nominal'). This too has some
reason to it, and examples can be seen in the literature. Fisher's
exact test is mathematically very complex and, even with modern
computer power, can take a long time to compute. The chi-square
test is an approximation of Fisher's exact test, which is based on a
very much simpler algebraic formula that can be computed in a
few moments with just a simple calculator. However, the scale is
specifically designed to have an ordering to it, and it is inefficient
to ignore this. Options A and D are better than B and E, but still not
optimal.

Option C is a 'non-parametric' test, which does not assume any
underlying distribution for the data but does take account of the
ordering across the scale points. There is a statistical problem in
that many observations will be the same (ie tied), but as the study is
described as 'small' this should not be a major concern. There is
no ideal analysis for this study, but option C makes the best use of
the data and the least dubious assumptions about the statistical
properties of the pain scale

**16.5   E: The range of values, 3.34–3.66 litres, excludes the population
mean with a probability of 0.05**

Confidence intervals relate to values of the population mean and
are usually expressed in terms of limits that include the population
mean with probability 0.95. Option E is stating this in a slightly
indirect way. Options A and B can be dismissed straight away as
the statements refer to subjects rather than the population mean.
Similarly, option C is a statement about the sample mean rather
than a statement about the population mean. Option D is incorrect
because limits for any variable need to be based on the
distribution of the individuals rather than on confidence intervals
for means.

INDEX